THE COMPLETE GLYCEMIC INDEX DIET FOR DIABETES

YOUR ESSENTIAL COMPANION TO LOW-GLYCEMIC DIET FOR DIABETES - WITH GI VALUES FOR OVER 3000 FOODS & FOOD LISTS FOR DIABETES

DR. H. MAHER

D1519761

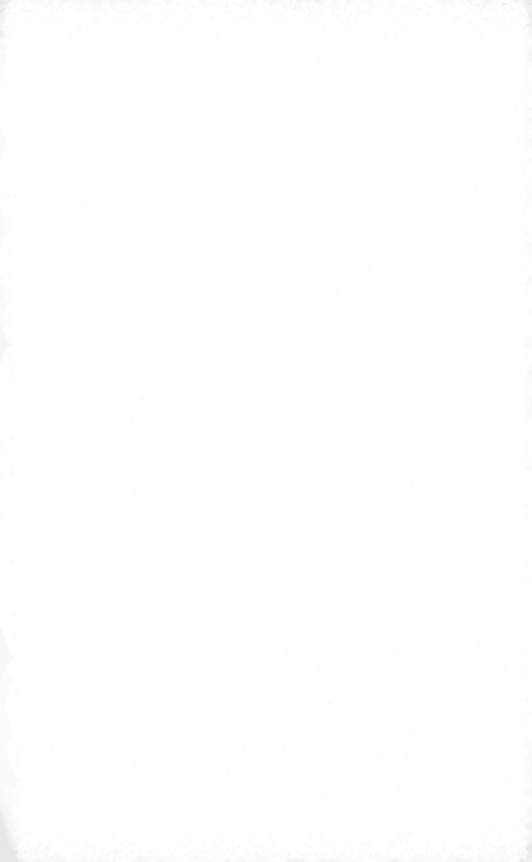

CONTENTS

INTRODUCTION

Diabetes is a chronic metabolic illness marked by unsuitable hyperglycemia due to a lack of insulin or insulin resistance. Its adverse health effects can significantly reduce life expectancy. Several lifestyle factors and dietary habits affect the incidence of type 1 and type 2 diabetes, such as types and amounts of food ingested, weight gain, obesity, physical activity, watching TV or sedentary time, sleep quality.

The glycemic index diet for diabetes is a targeted balanced diet with sufficient and right nutritional elements to battle diabetes, prevent diabetes complications, lower inflammation, improve mental health, and help you lose weight. Both nutritional deficiency and excess are tied with diseases and poor health conditions. Nutritional excess, particularly in highly-processed foods, refined carbohydrates, saturated fats, trans-fatty acids, sugar-sweetened foods, and sodium, can result in severe diabetes complications, poor glycemic control, cardiovascular disease, bone disorders, as well as obesity. In contrast, nutritional deficiencies can lead to impairments of body function, weight loss, fatigue, and conditions associated with vitamin and mineral deficiencies.

The primary foundation of the glycemic index diet for diabetes relies on the studies that established the strong relationship between what people eat and how it impacts their blood glucose level. In the past, carbohydrates were only classified according to their chemical structure as being either simple or complex. However, this division does not take into account the effects of carbohydrates on blood sugar, inflammation, and chronic diseases. The glycemic index (GI) system was developed to better categorize carbohydrate-containing foods. The GI system assigns values to foods based on how quickly and how high those foods cause spikes in blood glucose levels. Foods low on the glycemic index scale tend to release glucose in the blood slowly and steadily. In contrast, foods high on the glycemic index scale are quickly digested and absorbed and cause significant fluctuations in blood glucose.

The glycemic index ranks carbohydrates on a scale from 0 to 100:

- low glycemic foods comprise foods that have a rating of 55 or less
- medium glycemic foods comprise foods that have a rating in the range of 56 to 69
- high glycemic foods comprise foods that cause high spikes in blood sugar. Their glycemic index values are equal to or higher to 70

The reasoning behind the Glycemic index Diet for Diabetes is logical, strong and aims to select the foods that are considered low glycemic and avoid foods causing high fluctuations in blood sugar. Thus eating adequate portion sizes of low glycemic whole foods will result in better glycemic control, decreased inflammation, and reduced risk of diabetes complications.

Eating to lower the levels of blood sugar is not a one-size-fits-all approach. Different people, even twins, may respond to the same foods very differently. However, following the diabetic glycemic index dietary pattern will ensure you get the most of its beneficial effects. People who adhere to this diet more closely have consistently lower levels of blood sugar levels, lower blood pressure, increased LDL cholesterol, reduced HDL cholesterol, and reduced triglycerides than those following other diets. The Glycemic index Diet for Diabetes is considered healthier than modern fad diets (e.g., keto diet, low-carb, high-fat diets) because it is centered around eating low glycemic whole, unprocessed, or minimally processed foods and avoiding high glycemic foods and pro-inflammatory agents.

PART I

THE GLYCEMIC INDEX DIET
FOR DIABETES

1

DIABETES OVERVIEW

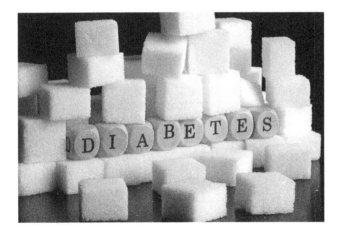

Diabetes is a chronic metabolic illness marked by unsuitable hyper-glycemia due to a lack of insulin or insulin resistance. Its adverse health effects can seriously reduce life expectancy significantly by ten years. Several lifestyle factors and dietary habits affect the incidence of type 1 and type 2 diabetes, such as types and amounts of food ingested, weight gain, obesity, physical activity, watching TV or sedentary time, sleep quality.

Diabetes mellitus refers to a chronic disease that influences how the body utilizes food for energy and is marked by abnormally high blood glucose levels. Insulin — the hormone made by the pancreas — allows glucose to get into body cells to provide energy. When blood sugar levels rise after eating, your pancreas releases a sufficient amount of insulin into the blood. Insulin then reduces blood sugar to keep it in the normal range. In people who have diabetes, the pancreas cannot perform this fundamental function, or the body's cells do not respond adequately to the produced insulin. The blood sugar level then increases, and sugar accumulates in the body and becomes toxic to the vital organs. Having a high glucose level in the blood can cause severe health problems. It can cause severe damages to the eyes, kidneys, heart, and nerves irreversibly.

Diabetes Mellitus is the most common chronic endocrine disorder caused mainly by inflammation according to recent high-quality research. There are three main types of diabetes:

- I. Type I diabetes

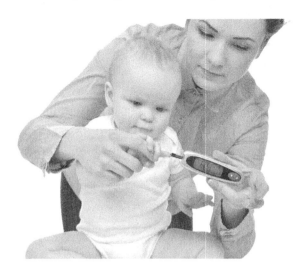

Type 1 diabetes is a chronic autoimmune disease characterized by the immune system's destruction of insulin-producing pancreatic *beta* cells. The body will no longer make insulin due to irreversible damages to the insulin-producing cells. Without insulin hormones, glucose can not get into the body's cells and the blood glucose increases above normal. People with type 1 must then inject daily insulin doses and follow a strict diet to stay alive and prevent the severe adverse effect. Type 1 diabetes generally appears in children and young adults but may occur at any age.

In 2016, the U.S. Food and Drug Administration (FDA) approved artificial pancreas to replace the manual blood glucose checking and the injection of insulin shots. These automated devices act like your real pancreas in controlling blood sugar and releasing insulin when the patient's blood sugar becomes too high. The artificial pancreas also releases a small flow of insulin continuously.

Symptoms of type 1 diabetes are serious and usually happen quickly, over a few days to weeks. Symptoms can include

- frequent thirst and urination
- increased hunger
- unexplained weight loss

- blurred vision
- frequent infections
- fatigue and tiredness

Unfortunately, type 1 diabetes is chronic immune-mediated and remains incurable. However, as you'll see in the chapter, "Vitamin D Optimal Doses", you will be able to improve the management of the disease significantly and prevent the development of diabetes-related chronic diseases.

- **2. Type 2 diabetes**

Prediabetes. Even if a person is not sick, he may suffer from prediabetes without knowing it. This term refers to an intermediate stage characterized by an abnormally higher blood glucose level than usual. That represents a warning signal that informs people with prediabetes diagnosis that they are at increased risk of type 2 diabetes mellitus if they don't take appropriate and urgent action, especially if they have other risk factors, including:

- overweight,
- obesity,
- sedentary lifestyle,
- high blood pressure.

In Type 2 diabetes, the mechanism is different from type 1 diabetes: insulin is normally secreted by the pancreas but with lower efficiency. Therefore, without sufficient insulin, the glucose stays in the blood. Type 2 diabetes is induced by several factors, including lifestyle factors, strict diets, overweight, obesity, Hyperthyroidism, and genes.

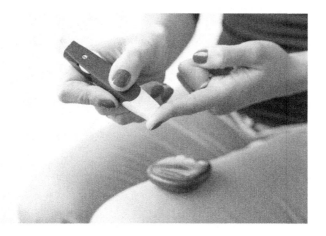

Type 2 diabetes can also develop at any age. However, it's more common after the age of forty.

- **3. Gestational diabetes**

Gestational diabetes is the high blood sugar that develops during pregnancy in women who did not have diabetes before becoming pregnant. Gestational diabetes is more frequent in the second or third trimester but can occur at any time of pregnancy and usually disappears after giving birth.

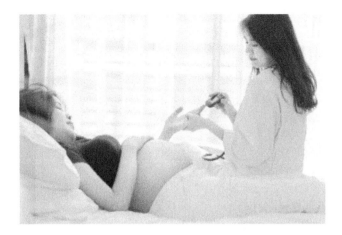

Women diagnosed with it are at higher risk of developing type 2 diabetes later in life, particularly for women with favoring factors (obesity, imbalanced diet, sedentary lifestyle, metabolic syndrome...).

Symptoms

Diabetes symptoms may vary depending on the level of blood sugar. Some people with prediabetes or type 2 diabetes may not experience frank symptoms at first. Conversely, with type 1 diabetes, symptoms come on quickly and severely.

Bellow a list of common symptoms and signs of type 1 and type 2 diabetes, and gestational diabetes:

- increased craving
- frequent urination
- excessive hunger
- weight loss
- ketones in urine
- fatigue and tiredness
- increased irritability
- blurred vision
- slow-healing wounds and cuts
- frequent infections

- **4. The A1C Test and Diabetes**

The A1C test (also called hemoglobin A1C or HbA1c test) is a blood test that measures the average levels of your blood sugar over the past two to three months. The A1C test is one of the commonly used tests to diagnose the risk of prediabetes or type 2 diabetes. The A1C test is the main tool for diabetes management, as patients use it to achieve their individual A1C goals.

How does the test work?

The A1C (HbA1c) test measures the amount of sugar in your blood that is attached to hemoglobin, a protein inside your red blood cells that carries oxygen. When sugar enters your bloodstream, it binds with hemoglobin. The A1C (HbA1c) test measures the percentage of your red blood cells that are coated with glucose. Thus, a higher A1C (HbA1c) level indicates poor blood glucose control and warns of an elevated risk of developing severe diabetes complications.

If you have a diabetes condition, you should get an A1C (HbA1c) test at least twice a year to make sure diabetes is under close control and your blood glucose is in your target range.

Interpreting the A1C results

A normal A1C (HbA1c) level is under 5.7%. In healthy people, the normal range for the A1c (HbA1c) level is in the range of 4% to 5.6%

A level of A1C (HbA1c) in the range of 5.7% to 6.4% indicates prediabetes and a higher chance of developing diabetes.

A level of A1C (HbA1c) equal to or high than 6.5% indicates diabetes.

2

ADHERING TO A HEALTHY LIFESTYLE

Over time, having an excess of sugar in your blood can cause complications ranging from mild to severe. Diabetes complications are often interrelated, share the same contributing causes, and combine in a dangerous way that may alter the overall health condition. For example, nearly 50% of all patients diagnosed with type 2 diabetes have high blood pressure (hypertension), which may constrict and narrow the blood vessels throughout the body, including the nerves, the eyes, and the kidney. On the other side, having high levels of glucose in your blood for a prolonged time can harm blood vessels that supply oxygen throughout your body, including the eyes, heart, kidneys, and brain. Damages that occur can lead to severe and long-term complications.

Diabetes also induces significant quantitative changes in the amount of circulating lipids characterized by an increase in triglycerides (a type of lipid in the blood), a reduction in HDL cholesterol (good), and an increase in LDL cholesterol (bad). These changes are associated with an increased risk of heart disease and stroke.

The main complications of diabetes

Diabetes complications are long-term problems that develop gradually. DM complications can lead to severe damage if untreated.

- diabetic retinopathy. People with diabetes are at risk of developing an eye disorder called retinopathy due to elevated high blood pressure. Retinopathy can affect patients' eyesight and cause partial vision loss and blindness.
- diabetic foot ulcers. Foot problems are severe diabetes complications that result from concomitant actions, including damages to the nerve and impaired blood circulation. Nerve damages known as diabetic neuropathy combined with reduced blood flow affect the feeling in your feet and make it difficult for sores and cuts to heal. In some serious cases, gangrenes develop and can lead to amputation.
- diabetic nephropathy. This severe diabetes complication is common among type 1 and types 2 diabetes patients who poorly control their blood glucose. Over time, uncontrolled diabetes can lead to irreversible damages to blood vessel clusters that filter waste and extra water out of your blood. This severe condition can lead to kidney damage and kidney failure. Your kidneys are also involved in the control of blood pressure, and such damages may cause hypertension which in turn worsen kidney diseases.
- heart disease and stroke. Over time, high blood glucose can harm blood vessels and nerves that control your heart and supply oxygen to the brain and heart. Individuals with diabetes are at higher risk of developing heart disease and strokes.
- erectile dysfunction. Poor and prolonged blood glucose control may damage nerves and small blood vessels that control the erection.
- chronic inflammatory diseases. Poorly controlled diabetes may cause damage to the whole body, trigger and worsen inflammation. In turn, inflammation causes and aggravates

insulin resistance leading to much-elevated blood glucose levels.

A healthy lifestyle

Adhering to the glycemic index diet for diabetes is more than selecting foods you eat, restricting your carbohydrates intake, and avoiding foods that cause high blood sugar spikes; it's also about sticking to the proper lifestyle that promotes better diabetes management, healthier life, and well-being. Thus, you have to focus simultaneously on your diet and lifestyle to reap all benefits of the glycemic index diet for diabetes and improve your blood sugar control.

You can only focus on diet and keep your habits, but you'll not experience optimum health and win your battle against diabetes. The two significant areas in which change is highly advised are physical activity and sleeping habits. Practicing regular physical activity will drive many beneficial effects in improving blood sugar control and insulin sensitivity. It will also help you prevent, delay, and reduce morbidities and complications associated with diabetes Mellitus. Sleeping well helps your body and brain function correctly, boost your immune system, improve your mental health, and can improve your diabetes management and prevent, or delay, diabetes complications. By committing to these easy and positive changes, you will expect to achieve better blood glucose control, positive health outcomes, and prevent diabetes complications.

Based on the best and latest science of how and what to eat, the diabetes glycemic index lifestyle is meant to be your global road map for managing diabetes, which is the key to preventing, reducing, or delaying complications. You are advised to use "ABCDEs of diabetes" as a way to manage your new diabetes glycemic index lifestyle:

- A- A stands for A1C, or HbA1c test, which assesses your blood glucose control over the past two to three months. So, get a regular A1C (HbA1c) test to measure your average blood glucose and target to stay under 7% as much as possible.
- B- B refers to blood pressure. Nearly half of people with type 2 diabetes suffer from hypertension. Try to keep your blood pressure below 130/80 mm Hg (or 140/90 mm Hg in some cases).
- C- C refers to cholesterol. Total blood cholesterol, HDL cholesterol (good), LDL cholesterol (bad), and triglycerides levels should be monitored. Your doctor will use the information and, if needed, develop a strategy to reduce your risks.
- D- D refers to diet. It refers to adhering to the glycemic index diet for diabetes and, if indicated, drug therapy. Your doctor may prescribe medicines that may help you lower your blood glucose, blood pressure (if applicable), cholesterol, and triglyceride levels (if applicable).
- E- E refers to exercice. You should practice regular physical activities for at least 150 minutes per week (e.g., 30 minutes, 6 days a week).

3

FOOD, WEIGHT LOSS AND DIABETES

Eating to lower the levels of blood sugar is not a one-size-fits-all approach. Different people, even twins, may respond to the same foods very differently. However, following the diabetic glycemic index dietary pattern will ensure you get the most of its beneficial effects. People who adhere to this diet more closely have consistently lower levels of blood sugar levels, lower blood pressure, increased LDL cholesterol, reduced HDL cholesterol, and reduced triglycerides than those following other diets. It is considered healthier than modern fad diets (e.g., keto diet, low-carb, high-fat diets) because it is centered around eating low glycemic whole, unprocessed, or minimally processed foods and avoiding high glycemic foods and pro-inflammatory agents.

- **Diet, Weight Loss, and Diabetes**

For years, hundreds of diets have been created with a lot of promises in terms of weight loss, inflammation reduction, diabetes reversal. Low-fat diets, low carb high fats diets were thought to be the best approaches to lose weight, control diabetes, and achieve a healthy weight. However, a growing body of evidence shows that these diets often don't work:

- low-fat diets have the tendency to replace fat with easily digested carbohydrates.
- low-carb high-fat diets overlook the importance of carbohydrates and often replace carbohydrates with highly processed fat-containing foods.
- fad diets often overlook the body's fundamental need for a balanced diet

The best diets, those that work, restrict calories to some extent, supply sufficient and high-quality nutrients, banish bad foods, and balance hormones that help lower your blood sugar, improve your glycemic control, and regulate your weight. Diets do this in three main ways:

1. getting you to eat sufficient good foods and/or banish bad ones
2. getting you aware of foods and nutrients you should include in your diet to achieve weight loss, better diabetes control, and prevent complications.
3. changing some of your bad eating habits and the ways you consider highly processed foods and refined carbohydrates

The best diet for losing weight and/or diabetes control is one that is good for all body parts, from your brain to your heart to your pancreas. It is also a diet you can embrace and live with for a long time. In other words, a powerful diet rooted in nature that offers a flexible eating pattern, provides healthy choices, banishes unhealthy foods, and doesn't require an extensive (and probably expensive) shopping list or supplements.

A diabetic balanced diet with sufficient and right nutritional elements is critical for battling diabetes, weight gain, and obesity. Both nutritional deficiency and excess are tied with diseases and poor health conditions. Nutritional excess, particularly in highly-processed foods, refined carbohydrates, saturated fats, trans-fatty acids, sugar-sweetened foods, and sodium, can result in severe chronic inflammatory illnesses such as autoimmune disease, cardio-vascular disease, bone disorders, diabetes as well as obesity. In contrast, nutritional deficiencies can lead to impairments of body function, weight loss, fatigue, and conditions associated with vitamin and mineral deficiencies.

One diet that allows that is a Low glycemic type diet. Such a diet—and its many variations—usually include:

- several servings of plant foods (e.g., vegetables, fruits) a day
- whole and minimally processed foods
- daily serving of seeds and nuts
- healthy fats and oils high in omega-3 fatty acids (canola, cod liver oil, fatty fish, flaxseed oil, Walnut oil, sunflower oil, etc.)
- lean protein mainly from fish, poultry, and nuts
- limited amounts of red meat
- limited amounts of sodium
- very limited quantities of refined carbohydrates (e.g., white flour, white, rice, white sugar, brown sugar, honey, corn syrup)
- limited alcoholic drinks
- NO high glycemic index foods
- NO trans fats
- NO highly processed foods

- **Dietary carbohydrates and diabetes**

Increased intake of carbohydrates-containing foods with a higher glycemic index is found to cause a high spike in blood sugar and insulin release, making it harder to control diabetes, increasing the risk of developing diabetes for healthy people, increasing the risk of severe complications, and worsening inflammation. Conversely, eating carbohydrates-containing foods with a low glycemic index is associated with positive health outcomes, including modulating inflammation, regulating immune system responses, and will help you gain close control over your blood sugar.

In addition, many studies have established that the quality of carbohydrates has a significant impact on inflammation, and the occurrence of diabetes complications. Low-quality carbohydrates such as highly processed foods and refined carbs are associated with increased inflammation, both acute and chronic, impaired immune system responses, poor blood glucose control, and increased risk of diabetes complications. Conversely, high-quality foods such as whole foods or minimally processed food with low glycemic index food are linked with better health outcomes, including better control of blood glucose, and reduced acute and chronic inflammation.

- **Dietary fats and diabetes**

Another important nutrient you should consider as part of a glycemic index diet for diabetes is fat. Eating the right amount of the right type of fat is essential whether you are managing diabetes or aiming to achieve a healthy weight.

In addition, fats are higher in calories per gram compared to proteins or carbohydrates. A gram of dietary fat has nearly 9 calories, while a gram of carbohydrate has roughly 4 calories or protein has about 4 calories. Thus, you should be aware of serving sizes when eating fats.

Eating the right types of fat is also critical for managing type 1 and type 2 diabetes and lowering the risk of developing some chronic diseases such as heart illnesses, strokes, kidneys diseases, and chronic inflammatory diseases.

Several studies have established that replacing trans fats and saturated fats with unsaturated fats (monounsaturated and polyunsaturated) reduces the risk of cardiovascular diseases in high-risk populations, including individuals with diabetes.

In addition, studies also found that replacing trans fats and saturated fat intake with low glycemic carbohydrates (e.g., wholegrain, fiber-rich fruits, fiber-rich vegetables, beans) results in cardiovascular benefits without altering the blood glucose control.

On the other side, a growing body of evidence has revealed how dietary fat intake affects the inflammatory status and focused on the gut microbiome as an important factor explaining the increase of inflammation biomarkers and fat intake. Trans fats are tied with various adverse health effects, worsen inflammation, and trigger some diabetes complications. The consumption of high amounts of saturated fats increases the LDL cholesterol (bad form) promotes and aggravates inflammation.

The American Diabetes Association recommends swapping saturated and trans fats in your diet by healthiest choices such as monounsaturated and polyunsaturated fats.

Healthy fats such as omega-3 fatty acids are associated with decreased inflammation and reduced risk of developing some chronic conditions. Several studies have investigated the role of omega-3 fatty acids in association with metformin to reduce triglyceride levels in diabetic patients with hypertriglyceridemia. Omega-3 fatty acids were found effective in reducing the triglyceride level significantly by 20-65%. Omega-3 fatty acids were also found to improve the effectiveness of statins and thus decrease the risk of cardiovascular diseases among diabetic patients with hypertriglyc-eridemia.

- **The Essential Role of Vitamin D**

It is established that Vitamin D is essential for normal glucose metabolism and improvement of insulin sensitivity. Therefore, vitamin D supplementation appears to promote glucose-mediated insulin secretion allowing vitamin D to play a beneficial role in glucose metabolism by:

1. regulating insulin secretion and promoting the survival of beta-cells, which results in releasing insulin in a tightly regulated manner to maintain blood glucose levels in the adequate range.
2. regulating the calcium flux within beta-cells, which results in improving insulin secretion directly because insulin secretion is a calcium-dependent process. Vitamin D stimulates insulin secretion and benefits beta-cell secretory function when calcium levels are adequate.
3. modulating the adaptive and innate immune responses which results in a preventative effect on autoimmune such as type 1 diabetes. Vitamin D modulates the immune system's response and prevents the destruction of insulin-secreting pancreatic beta-cells, which causes the development of type 1 diabetes.
4. reducing substantially systemic inflammation involved in insulin resistance and the development of type 2 diabetes. Recent studies have established that vitamin D plays an essential role in modulating the inflammation system by inhibiting the proliferation of pro-inflammatory cells and regulating the production of inflammatory cytokines.

5. improving insulin sensitivity and enhancing pancreatic beta-cell function.

4

THE GLYCEMIC INDEX DIET EXPLAINED

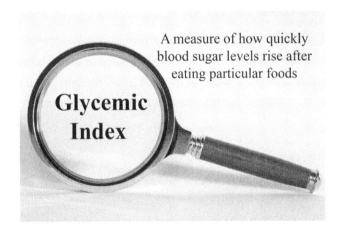

- **The Glycemic Index Diet**

The glycemic index (GI) was initially developed in the early 1980s to scientifically determine how different foods containing carbohydrates — vegetables, legumes, fruits, processed foods, and dairy products — affect blood sugar levels. Since that initial research led by Dr. Jenkins took place more than 35 years ago, many scientists identified the opportunity that the glycemic index could be a powerful tool for maintaining weight, improving effective weight-loss diets, and managing diabetes.

The glycemic index isn't formally a diet in the sense that you have to conform to strict rules, follow particular meal plans or eliminate some foods from your daily meals. Instead, it's a scientific method of identifying how carbohydrates in foods affect blood sugar levels and measuring how slowly or quickly the carbohydrates in foods raise blood sugar. Thus, the Glycemic Index referential is particularly important to know if you want to maintain weight, lose weight or if you're going to take more control of diabetes and specific health issues.

The "glycemic index (GI) diet" refers to a targeted diet plan that uses the glycemic index as the primary and only guides for meal planning. Unlike other diet plans that provide strict recommendations, the glycemic index diet doesn't specify the daily amount of calories, carbohydrates, protein, or fats for weight maintenance or weight loss. Still, it provides an effective eating plan with more flexibility and sustainable results in terms of weight loss, weight management, diabetes control, and inflammation-healing and prevention.

- **Understanding GI values**

Glycemic index (GI) values are divided into three categories:

- Low GI: This category comprises foods that have their GI value below 55
- Medium GI: This category comprises foods that have their GI value in the range 56 to 69
- High GI: In general, this category must be avoided because foods cause high spikes in the blood sugar level. Their GI value are equal or higher to 70

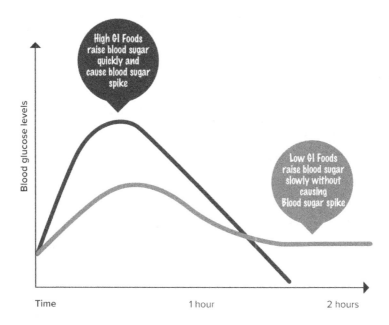

Comparing the GI values may help guide your food choices. For example, muesli has a GI value of 86 ± 4. A Smoothie drink, a banana has a GI value of 30 ± 4.

- **How does Glycemic Index (GI) Diet work?**

Eating according to the Glycemic Index Diet looks simple, because all you need to know is where different foods fall on the 0 to 100 glycemic index (GI).

- You fill up on low GI foods (GI value: 55 and under)
- Eat smaller amounts of medium GI foods (GI value:56 to 69)
- And mostly avoid high GI foods (GI value: 70 and up)

Lists of foods in the 14 categories are available in this book:

- Beef, Lamb, Veal, Pork & Poultry
- Beverages
- Bread & Bakery Products
- Breakfast Cereals
- Dairy Products & Alternatives
- Soups, Pasta, and Noodles
- Fish & Fish Products
- Fruit and Fruit Products
- Legumes and Nuts
- Meat Sandwiches and Ham
- Mixed Meals and Convenience Foods
- Recipe
- Snack Foods and Confectionery
- Vegetables

Besides referring to these lists as needed, there is no difficult weighing or measuring and no need to track your calories intake. However, you will have to concoct your eating plan and menus yourself.

- **How Is Glycemic Index Measured?**

Glycemic Index values of foods are measured using valid and proven scientific methods and cannot be guessed just by looking at the composition of specific food or the nutrition facts on food packaging.

Thus, the GI calculation follows the international standard method and provides values that are commonly accepted. The Glycemic Index value of food is calculated by feeding over ten healthy people a portion of the food object of the study and containing fifty grams of digestible carbohydrate and then measuring the effect for each participant on his blood glucose levels (blood glucose response) over the next two hours.

The second part of the process consists of giving the same participants an equal carbohydrate portion of the glucose (used as the reference food) and measuring their blood glucose response over the next two hours.

The Glycemic Index value for the food is then calculated for each participant by using a simple formula (dividing the blood glucose response for the food by their blood glucose response for the glucose (reference food)). The final value of the Glycemic Index for the food is the average Glycemic Index value for the participants (over 10).

Carbohydrates with a low GI value (55 or less) are more slowly digested, absorbed, and metabolized and cause a smaller and slower rise in blood glucose and, therefore, usually, insulin levels.

A low glycemic diet or foods are associated with reduced risks of chronic disease. Foods that have a low glycemic index are known for their property to release glucose in the blood slowly and regularly. Conversely, Foods that have a high glycemic index are known for their property to release glucose rapidly. Researches suggest that foods with a low glycemic index (LGI foods) are ideal for weight loss diets and foster lasting weight loss, in addition to their positive effect on the pancreas (insulin release), eyes, and kidney.

* **The Glycemic Load Concept**

Basing your food choices only on the GI means that you're focusing on only one aspect of the food and ignoring other important aspects, such as the quality and quantity of the carbohydrates in the foods. Here comes the importance of the glycemic load, which combines the two criteria and provides, when available, an additional tool for better weight loss control and effective diabetes management.

Glycemic Load was introduced later to fill the gap and represents another critical tool to track carbohydrates quality and quantity.

Glycemic Load (GL) combines both the quality and amount of carbohydrates following a simple formula:

**Glycemic Load (GL) = GI x Carbohydrate (grams) content per
portion ÷ 100**

For example, an apple that has a GI of 32 and contains 13 grams of
carbohydrates is considered as more healthier than Sweet potato that
has a GL of 11 using the glycemic load tool.

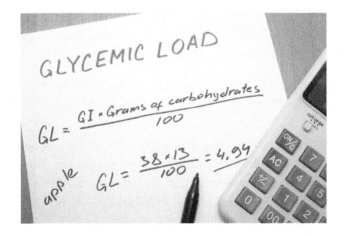

Like the glycemic index, the glycemic load (GL) of a food can be classified as:

- **Low:** 10 or less
- **Medium:** 11 – 19
- **High:** 20 or more

Should I use the GI or the GL?

There's no need for you to calculate or track the glycemic index (GL)
of your meals. Although the concept of glycemic load (GL) has been
useful and well documented in scientific research, it's the glycemic

index (GI) that is proven most helpful and powerful to people who are overweight and those with diabetes.

If you use the glycemic index (GI) as it was initially intended –to choose the lower glycemic index (GI) food within a meal group or food category– you will then be selecting the one with the lowest glycemic load (GL) value provided you eat an adequate portion. The classification of food in nutrition is pertinent, and foods are grouped following the main principle –they contain similar nutrients (carbohydrate, protein, fat, vitamins) and include comparable amounts of carbohydrates. Then, choosing healthy foods according to their low GI values, at least one at each meal, chances are you are following an eating plan that not only keeps your blood glucose at the safest levels but contains balanced amounts of essential nutrients –carbohydrates, proteins, and fats. To help you lower your blood sugar, the portions sizes of different foods are given in chapter II "Meal Planning Guidelines"

5
THE HEALTH BENEFITS OF THE LOW GLYCEMIC DIET

Lowering your insulin levels is one of the secrets to better glycemic control and management, lasting weight loss, and improved health conditions. High insulin levels caused by eating high glycemic index foods are harmful and promote long-term high blood fat, high blood glucose, and high blood pressure and increase the risk of a heart attack. Because of this, following the low GI diet is beneficial in controlling your blood sugar level, driving weight loss in the mid and long-term, preventing diabetes, PCOS, and heart disease, and improving your overall health.

Unlike other popular low-carbohydrates, high protein diets, eating a low glycemic index diet has been scientifically proven to help people:

- control blood sugar and lower insulin release
- reduce the risk of developing type 2 diabetes
- improve women's gestational diabetes management and reduce adverse pregnancy outcomes
- prevent diabetes complications
- achieve and maintain a healthy weight
- reduce PCOS symptoms

- maintain a healthy condition
- reduce significantly the risk of developing metabolic syndrome
- prevent heart attack and stroke

Low-glycemic index diet and Insulin Resistance Reversal

Insulin resistance is a serious and silent health condition that occurs when cells in your muscles, liver, and body fat start ignoring the signal that insulin hormone is sending out to transfer sugar out of the bloodstream and put it into your body cells. As insulin resistance develops, the body reacts by producing more and more insulin to lower blood sugar.

Over time, the β cells in the pancreas working hard to make a higher supply of insulin can no longer provide more and more insulin. Your blood sugar then reflects the pancreas' failure to maintain the level in the healthy range, and your blood sugar rises, showing prediabetes or, at worst, diabetes type 2.

Insulin resistance is silent and presents no symptoms in the first stage of its development. The symptoms appear later when the condition worsens, and the pancreas cannot produce enough insulin to keep your blood sugar within the normal range. When this occurs, the symptoms may be severe including, metabolic syndrome, polycystic ovary syndrome (PCOS), and various types of diabetes.

Fortunately, it is possible to reduce the effects of insulin resistance and boost your insulin sensitivity by following a low-glycemic index diet.

High glycemic index foods affect your weight and health.

Consuming high glycemic index foods may be harmful to your health and causes high spikes of your blood sugar compared to low glycemic index foods as shown in the following figure.

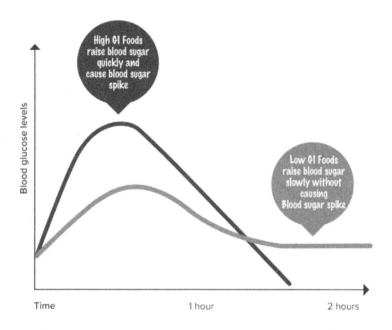

High glycemic food consumption has also been associated with an increased risk of diabetes complications, a higher risk of obesity, insulin resistance, fatty liver, metabolic syndrome, and an elevated risk of chronic disease.

Low-glycemic index Diet is Better for Your Body

Carbohydrates found in natural foods, such as legumes, fruits, vegetables, meats, fish, and grains, tend to be more complex and harder to digest, and had generally low-glycemic index values. Eating such foods will lead to smooth increases and falls in your blood glucose levels, which help you improve your overall health, prevent obesity, help diabetes control, and prevent diabetes complications.

Following a low glycemic diet may provide several health benefits, including:

- diabetes management (gestational diabetes, type I and type 2 diabetes)
- long-lasting weight loss,
- obesity control,
- reduction of heart strokes
- prevention of coronary heart disease
- PCOS prevention

Low-glycemic index diet leads to hunger-reduction

Leptin, referred to as the starvation or "hunger hormone," is a hormone produced by fat tissues and is secreted into our bloodstream. It plays an essential role in weight regulation by reducing a person's appetite.

Eating low-glycemic-index foods translates to eating foods that lower the insulin response and increase circulating leptin levels inducing a post-meal condition favorable for reduced food consumption due to a lower person's appetite. This may be very beneficial in such situations:

- type 2 diabetes management
- obesity control
- weight loss
- weight maintenance management
- insulin resistance

When you eat the right foods, you will notice that your appetite is under control due to the leptin effect. Your insulin levels will also be more stabilized, and your sugar levels will rise and falls smoothly.

6

CARB COUNTING AND GLYCEMIC INDEX

It is well established now that both the amount and the type of carbohydrate in food affect blood sugar levels. The total amount of carbohydrates in food was believed to provide a good prediction of the blood glucose response. Thus, eating fifty grams of pure sugar would cause the same blood glucose response as any fifty-gram carbohydrates-containing food. Which is completely wrong!!!

Because the quality of carbohydrates matters and does have a significant effect on blood glucose, using the glycemic index (GI) may be very helpful in tightly managing blood glucose. In other words, carbohydrate counting is essential but not sufficient, and you'll gain more control of diabetes management using this powerful tool (GI) and make smarter food choices.

In fact, carbohydrates in the food you ingest will raise your blood glucose levels. How fast they raise your blood glucose depends on the quality of the carbs and what you eat with them. For example, sugar levels in fruit or vegetable juice induce a notable spike in blood sugar levels, while sugar in the whole fruits or vegetables is digested more slowly. Carbohydrates-containing foods will be slowly digested if consumed with fat, fiber, or protein, thus inducing smoother increases in blood sugar levels.

Foods that contain glucose can be part of your diabetes dietary plan, provided they do not cause high spikes of blood sugar. You have then to rely on the glycemic index scale that provides valuable information on how each food affects blood sugar.

Types of Carbohydrates in Your Diet

When you eat carbohydrates, your body breaks them down into glucose (blood sugar), which are absorbed into the bloodstream. As the glucose level rises in your body, the pancreas releases insulin, a peptide hormone responsible for maintaining normal blood glucose levels. Insulin moves glucose from the blood into the cells, where it can be used as an energy source. Dietary carbohydrates can be divided into three major categories:

- Sugars: Short-chain carbs found in foods such as fructose, glucose, sucrose, and galactose.
- Starches: Long-chain of glucose molecules, which get transformed into glucose during digestion.
- Fibers: are divided into soluble and insoluble.

Carbohydrates can also be divided according to their chemical composition into simple and complex carbs:

- Complex carbohydrates are formed by sugar molecules that are linked together in complex and long chains. Complex carbs are found in vegetables, fruits, peas, beans, and whole grains and contain natural fiber. These types of food are healthy.
- Simple carbohydrates are transformed quickly by the body and induce an increased sugar blood level. They are found in high amounts in processed foods and refined sugars. The consumption of this type of carbs is associated with health

problems like type 2 diabetes, obesity, metabolism problem. Simple carbs foods are also deprived of essential nutrients and vitamins.

Choosing the best carbohydrate-containing foods

The quality of the carbohydrates you eat is crucial in adjusting the level of some hormones that influences diabetes, inflammation or controls weight gain, including insulin, cortisol, leptin, peptide YY. For instance, frequently eating low-quality carbs (high glycemic foods) will lead to frequent blood sugar spikes, which will:

- let controlling your blood sugar levels hard,
- promote or worsen inflammation,
- cause weight gain, obesity,
- cause insulin resistance for healthy individuals
- dysregulate cortisol levels.

Conversely, the soluble and insoluble fibers in whole foods (low glycemic foods) are known to offset glucose conversion, prevent higher insulin supplies, and avoid irregular blood sugar variations that induce an excess of cortisol and insulin release.

Estimating Portion Sizes Using Your Hand

PORTION SIZE

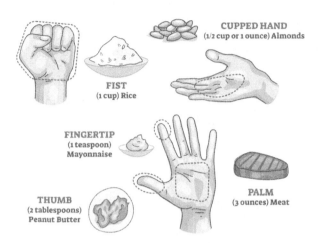

CUPPED HAND
(1/2 cup or 1 ounce) Almonds

FIST
(1 cup) Rice

FINGERTIP
(1 teaspoon)
Mayonnaise

THUMB
(2 tablespoons)
Peanut Butter

PALM
(3 ounces) Meat

This portion size measuring guide will help you estimate the amount of food on the plate without having to measure your portions.

The Palm

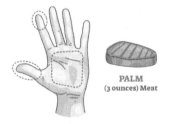

PALM
(3 ounces) Meat

The palm of your hand as shown in this figure may be used to estimate your protein intake. 1 palm is equivalent to a 3 ounces (oz.) serving of protein.

Examples of what you could estimate a 3-ounce serving include poultry, beef, fish, pork, and chicken.

The fist

A fist-sized portion is a great way of estimating a portion size of carbohydrates. You can use your fist to measure your intake of vegetables, fruits, cereals, and grains. I fist is equivalent to I cup.

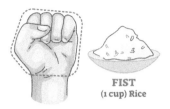

FIST
(1 cup) Rice

Tip of Thumb

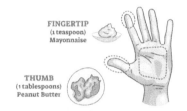

FINGERTIP
(1 teaspoon)
Mayonnaise

THUMB
(1 tablespoons)
Peanut Butter

The tip of a thumb is a great tool to estimate a portion size of healthy fat. You can use your tip of the thumb to estimate your fat intakes such as peanut butter, cheese, homemade salad dressings, butter. I thumb is equivalent to I tablespoon.

The fingertip

The fingertip is used to estimate the amount of healthy oils or fats you would consume. You can use your fingertip to measure your fat intakes such as nut butter, olive oil, homemade salad dressings, butter. I fingertip is equivalent to I teaspoon.

A Cupped Hand

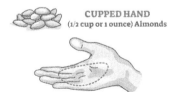

CUPPED HAND
(1/2 cup or 1 ounce) Almonds

The cupped hand is used to measure the amount of some foods such as nuts and seeds you would consume. You can use the surface area of your cupped hand to estimate a portion of seeds and nuts for example. I hand cupped is equivalent to a 1/2 cup.

7

EATING LOW GLYCEMIC AND ANTI-INFLAMMATORY FOODS

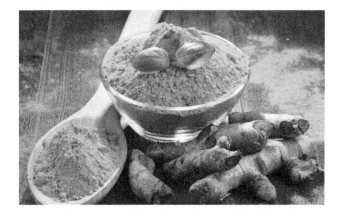

Growing lines of evidence indicate that various dietary polyphenols and flavonoids positively influence blood sugar at different levels, help control and prevent diabetes complications. Antioxidants also play a beneficial and protective role of the pancreatic beta-cells against glucose toxicity in diabetic patients. Thus, consuming polyphenols-rich foods, flavonoids-rich foods, and antioxidants will help you closely control your blood sugar levels, reduce the risk of developing chronic inflammatory diseases and prevent diabetes complications.

- **1. Eating low glycemic index vegetables and fruits**

In the glycemic index diet for diabetes, you have to eat low glycemic index fruits and vegetables to keep close control of your blood sugar level. In addition, non-starchy vegetables and fruits are good sources of anti-inflammatory nutrients such as polyphenols, antioxidants, and flavonoids which contribute to lowering inflammation and, in turn, reducing the risk of diabetes complications.

The serving sizes for low glycemic index vegetables and fruits are equivalent to:

- 1 cup raw or salad vegetables
- 1/2 cup cooked vegetables
- 3/4 cup (6oz) vegetable juice homemade and unsweetened
- ½ cup of cooked beans, lentils, and peas
- 1 medium piece of fruit
- 1 cup (6 oz) of sliced fruits
- ½ cup (4 oz) of fruit juice

The total vegetable intake (per day) is equivalent to 8-10 servings. You have to vary your meals using the maximal recommended amount as follows:

- "Dark-Green Vegetables" group up to 2 servings
- "Red & Orange Vegetables" group up to 3 servings
- "Beans, Peas, Lentils" group up to 2 servings
- "Starchy Vegetables" group up to 1 serving
- "Other Vegetables" group up to 3 servings

The total fruit intake is equivalent to 2-4 servings per day.

- **2. Increasing your Omega-3 Fatty Acids intake**

Omega-3 fatty acids are a healthy type of polyunsaturated fats associated with beneficial health effects such as

- decreasing inflammation
- improving heart health
- supporting mental health
- decreasing liver fat
- helping in the prevention of many chronic conditions
- promoting bone health

Strategies to increase your weekly intake of omega-3 fatty acids include regularly eating omega-3-rich nuts and seeds—such as chia seed, flaxseed, Hemp seed—, eating fatty fish—such as salmon, sardines, anchovies, mackerel, and herring. The weekly fish intake is equivalent to 10 servings (a serving is equal to 3 to 4 ounces). So target eating 6-8 servings of fatty fish per week.

- **3. Choosing healthy fats**

The glycemic index diet for diabetes is rich in omega-3 and lower in omega-6 than most diets. High levels of omega-3 combined with a low (omega-6/omega-3) are associated with many health benefits, including a significant reduction of unnecessary inflammation and diabetes complications. For example, a ratio (omega-6/omega-3) of 4/1 was correlated to a 70% reduction in mortality. So, based on recent studies, you have to keep the ratio (omega-6/omega-3) in the range of 1/1 and 4/1, which is associated with positive health outcomes.

Strategies to achieve an adequate ratio (omega-6/omega-3) include

- consuming fatty fish (e.g., sardines, mackerels, salmon, herring, anchovies) twice a week,
- consuming nuts and seeds (e.g., flax seeds, chia seeds, walnuts) twice a week.

- **4. Increasing olive oil consumption**

Recent studies have established that an extra virgin olive oil-rich diet reduces glucose levels, LDL cholesterol (bad), and triglycerides. And thus, prevents a series of illnesses that are very common among diabetic patients.

The anti-diabetes benefits of Extra Virgin Olive Oil (EVOO) increase with the daily ingested amount. A minimum of extra virgin olive oil of four tablespoons per day is necessary to provide beneficial anti-diabetes and antioxidant effects. When cooking, EVOO is an excellent choice as it has been well established that it helps reduce blood sugar levels, reduce blood pressure, lower bad cholesterol (LDL), and decrease inflammation. The nutritional composition of virgin olive is comprised of mainly

- monounsaturated fatty acids (69.2% for extra virgin olive oil), mainly Oleic acid (omega-9)
- saturated fats (15.4% for extra virgin olive oil) mainly Stearic acid and Palmitic Acid
- polyunsaturated (9.07% for extra virgin olive oil), mainly Linoleic acid (omega-3)
- Polyphenols
- Vitamin E, Carotenoids, and Squalene

Strategies to increase your daily intake of olive oil include

- replacing butter with EVOO,

- using olive oil as finishing oil for your meals,
- replacing the oil you use for cooking,
- roasting, and frying with EVOO.

- **5. Including anti-inflammatory spices in your eating plan**

Over the several last decades, extensive research has revealed that some spices and their active components exhibit tremendous anti-inflammatory benefits. Thus, spices have been found to prevent or decrease the severity of diabetes complications as well as a number of chronic conditions such as arthritis, asthma, multiple sclerosis, cardiovascular diseases, lupus, cancer, and neurodegenerative diseases. The most common spices used for their anti-inflammatory activities are

- turmeric,
- green tea,
- garlic,
- ginger,
- cayenne pepper,
- black pepper,
- black cumin,
- clove,
- cumin,
- ginseng,
- cardamom,
- parsley
- cinnamon,
- rosemary,
- chives,
- basil,
- cilantro

In addition, spices have a unique property to add flavor to any meal without adding fats or salt. Therefore, you should consider integrating herbs as part of your daily diet when cooking.

Some strategies for getting more herbs and spices in your diet include

- using some fresh herbs as the main ingredient (e.g., herb salad, tabbouleh salad),
- replacing some green vegetables in salads with herbs,
- substituting (or reducing) salt in a recipe with spices,
- replacing mayonnaise with basil-olive oil preparation,
- drinking 3–4 cups of green tea daily.

- **6. Drinking more water**

Water is critical for life. Without water, there is no life. All of the organs of our body, such as the heart, brain, lungs, and muscles, contain a significant quantity of water and need water to stay healthy.

Every day we lose water, and we need to replace it through a regular water supply. Otherwise, we can suffer from dehydration, which may alter the normal body's functions.

The recommended water intake for men aged 19+ is 3 liters (13 cups), and for women aged 19+ is 2.2 liters (9 cups) each day.

8

AVOIDING HIGH GLYCEMIC AND INFLAMMATORY FOODS

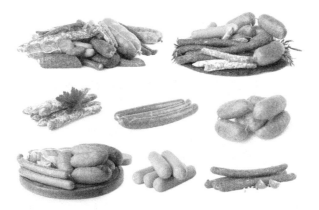

- **1. Limiting moderate glycemic index foods and avoiding high glycemic foods**

Eating according to the Glycemic Index Diet looks simple because all you need to know is where different foods fall on the 0 to 100 glycemic index (GI).

- You fill up on low glycemic index foods (GI value: 55 and

under)

- Eat smaller amounts of moderate glycemic index foods (GI value:56 to 69)
- And mostly avoid high glycemic index foods (GI value: 70 and up)

Tables of foods with their glycemic index divided into the 14 categories are available in part II, "Glycemic Index Counter":

- Beef, Lamb, Veal, Pork & Poultry
- Beverages
- Bread & Bakery Products
- Breakfast Cereals
- Dairy Products & Alternatives
- Soups, Pasta, and Noodles
- Fish & Fish Products
- Fruit and Fruit Products
- Legumes and Nuts
- Meat Sandwiches and Ham
- Mixed Meals and Convenience Foods
- Recipe
- Snack Foods and Confectionery
- Vegetables

- **2. Excluding Trans-Fats containing Foods**

Trans-fatty acids are mostly industrially manufactured fats produced during the hydrogenation process that adds hydrogen to liquid vegetable oils to transform the liquid to a solid form at room temperature. Trans fats give foods a desirable taste and texture. However, unlike other dietary fats, consuming trans-fatty acids raises the level of your bad cholesterol (LDL), lowers your good cholesterol (HDL) levels, increases your risk of developing severe cardiovascular conditions certain cancers, and aggravates inflammation. Trans fats may be present in several food products, including:

- fried fast foods, including french fries, fried chicken, battered fish, mozzarella sticks, and doughnuts
- margarine
- peanut butter
- baked goods, such as cakes, pies, and cookies made with margarine or vegetable shortening
- vegetable shortening

Strategies to reduce drastically trans fats intake include

- avoiding or reducing intakes of fried fast foods—including french fries, fried chicken, battered fish, mozzarella sticks, and doughnuts—margarine, peanut butter, frozen pizza, baked goods made with margarine or vegetable shortening
- eating smaller portion sizes
- consuming trans-fat-containing foods less frequently.

- **3. Eating a little less red meat but enough proteins**

There is little evidence that red meat may contribute to inflammation and alter glycemic control, while some recent studies revealed that unprocessed red meat might be associated with less inflammation and is safe for people with diabetes. However, there is a consensus about the danger of consuming processed red meat such as sausage, bacon, salami, and hot dogs. A 2012 study funded and supported by some health and nutrition government agencies has established the link between processed red meal consumption and increased total mortality. It also revealed that daily unprocessed red meat consumption raised the risk of total mortality by 13%. The study revealed that replacing one serving of red meat per day with other proteins sources such as fish, poultry, and nuts could decrease the risk of mortality by 7-19%.

These findings suggest that you should restrict your red meat intake to reduce inflammation, prevent and delay diabetes complications.

Eating an adequate amount of protein is extremely important for your health because proteins play a crucial role in your body's vital processes and metabolisms, such as building and repairing tissues, building muscles, blood, hair, and skin, regulating some inflammatory response, and producing hormones, enzymes, and other body chemicals. The weekly recommended proteins intake is equivalent to

- 30 servings of animal proteins (mainly lean white meat, and eggs)
- 10 servings of seafood
- 5 servings of nuts and seeds

By restricting red meat intake in the range of 1/5 to 1/4 of animal proteins (e.g., 6 to 7.5 servings of red meat per week), you may experience improvement in your overall health and reduction of some symptoms caused by inflammation.

9

EATING WHOLE AND MINIMALLY PROCESSED FOODS

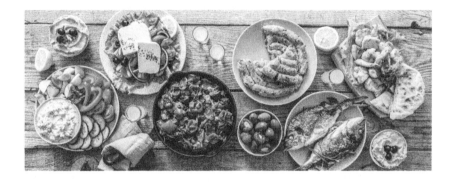

Most Americans don't eat whole foods anymore. They eat processed and highly-processed foods that are generally inferior to unprocessed or minimally processed foods. In fact, highly-processed foods are generally industrially-made and contain many ingredients, including high-fructose corn syrup, trans fats, monosodium glutamate, artificial sweeteners, flavors, colors, and other chemical additives. Highly-processed foods are believed to be a significant contributor to the obesity epidemic in the world, promoting diabetes, chronic inflammation, and the prevalence of autoimmune diseases. Therefore, we must distinguish between healthy processed foods to include in the glycemic index diet for diabetes and those to exclude because they are considered unhealthy and pro-inflammatory. For this reason, the next chapter (chapter 10) is fundamental because it contains foods groups based on the NOVA classification system. To adhere to the glycemic index diet for diabetes, you must get familiar with the four NOVA foods groups.

Whole food refers to unprocessed or minimally processed food— a nature-made food without added sugars, fat, sodium, flavorings, or other artificial ingredients. It has not been broken down by the man intervention into its components and refined into a new form. Whole Foods are generally close to their natural state, unprocessed and unrefined. Whole foods have little to no additives or preservatives.

A glycemic index diet for diabetes is not a specific diet. Instead, it refers to an eating plan that primarily selects low glycemic and whole foods and provides many health benefits, including better glycemic control, diabetes complication prevention, inflammation reduction, and hypertension prevention and treatment.

- **The glycemic index diet for diabetes main principles**

The glycemic index diet for diabetes is a revolutionary balanced, easy, long-term, and sustainable diet that selects low glycemic whole, minimally processed foods and limits animal products. It mainly focuses on plants, including vegetables, fruits, whole grains, legumes, seeds, and nuts, which should make up most of what you eat. You then have to design your eating plan around **unprocessed and mini-mally processed foods (NOVA group 1 of foods)** and, as much as you can, **avoid those that are processed (NOVA group 2 of foods)** and **absolutely exclude highly-processed (NOVA group 3 of foods)**.

The glycemic index diet for diabetes supplies your body with low glycemic unprocessed or minimally processed foods (**NOVA group 1 of foods**), with little to no unhealthy added constituents. You don't have to be focused on calorie, protein, fat, or carb counting. Instead, you have to concentrate on eating foods that do not cause high blood sugar spikes and battle inflammation.

The importance of the glycemic index component is critical because one can adopt a whole foods diet and still end up eating unhealthy carbohydrates-containing foods or fatty foods. Merely avoiding processed and refined foods is not the answer to better glycemic control, diabetes complications prevention, and inflammation reduction. Frequently eating carbohydrates-containing foods that cause high spikes in your blood sugar may make it harder to control your blood sugar and put you at increased risk of diabetes complications.

Coconut, coconut oil, palm kernel oil, and palm oil are fall in the category of whole foods but are full of saturated fats. Many experts, including the American Diabetes Association, the American Heart Association, claim that replacing foods high in saturated fat with healthier alternatives may lower LDL cholesterol and triglycerides in the blood. In addition, oils rich in saturated fats are associated with increased inflammation and chronic diseases.

Thus the glycemic index component is critical to address such problems and provide a robust solution to win against diabetes.

Carbohydrates, Proteins, and Fats: How do macronutrients fit into the glycemic index diet for diabetes?

1. Carbohydrates

The choice of high-quality macronutrients is crucial for the success of the glycemic index diet for diabetes.

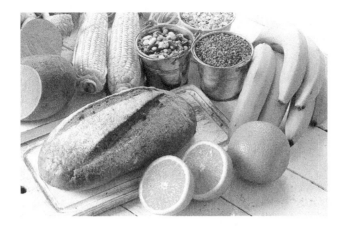

- **Knowing how carbohydrates can work for you or against you**

Eating a glycemic index diet for diabetes isn't just about eating unprocessed and minimally processed foods; a large part of controlling your blood glucose is strongly impacted by the type of carbohydrates you eat. All carbohydrates, whether they are low glycemic, moderate glycemic, or high glycemic, follow the same metabolic mechanism and break down into blood sugar, which plays a crucial role in the ability of our bodies to function properly. The problem with blood sugar and consequently with carbohydrates occurs when the blood sugar levels spike high throughout the day and frequently.

In response to these fast and large spikes in blood glucose, the pancreas releases a large amount of insulin which may induce insulin resistance, trigger and worsen inflammation.

Types of Carbohydrates in Your Diet

When you eat carbohydrates, your body breaks them down into glucose, which is absorbed into the bloodstream. As the glucose level rises in your body, the pancreas releases insulin, a peptide hormone responsible for maintaining normal blood glucose levels. Insulin moves glucose from the blood into the cells, where it can be used as an energy source. Dietary carbohydrates can be divided into three major categories:

- sugars: Short-chain carbs found in foods such as fructose, glucose, sucrose, and galactose.
- starches: Long-chain of glucose molecules, which get transformed into glucose during digestion.
- fibers: are divided into soluble and insoluble.

Carbohydrates can also be divided according to their chemical composition into simple and complex carbs:

- complex carbohydrates are formed by sugar molecules that are linked together in complex and long chains. Complex carbs are found in vegetables, fruits, peas, beans, and whole grains and contain natural fiber. These types of food are considered healthy.
- simple carbohydrates are transformed quickly by the body and induce blood sugar spikes. They are found in high amounts in processed foods and refined sugars. The consumption of this type of carbs is associated with medical conditions such as type 2 diabetes, obesity, metabolism problem. Simple carbs foods are also deprived of essential nutrients and vitamins.

Choosing the best carbohydrate-containing foods

The quality of the carbohydrates you eat is crucial in adjusting the level of some hormones that influences inflammation or controls weight gain, including insulin, cortisol, leptin, peptide YY. For instance, low-quality carbs (high glycemic foods) are quickly digested and lead to blood glucose spikes, which may aggravate diabetes, worsen inflammation, cause weight gain, obesity, insulin resistance, and increased cortisol levels. Conversely, the soluble and insoluble fibers in whole foods (low glycemic foods) are known to offset glucose conversion, prevent higher insulin supplies, and avoid irregular blood sugar variations that induce an excess of cortisol and insulin release.

2. Protein

Eating an adequate amount of protein is extremely important for your health because it plays a crucial role in your body's vital processes and metabolisms, such as building and repairing tissues, building muscles, blood, hair, and skin, and producing hormones, enzymes, and other body chemicals.

Unlike carbohydrates and fat, your body does not store protein, and you need to eat the necessary amount to keep the right hormonal balance and a healthy body.

Plus, eating protein reduces levels of ghrelin (the hunger hormone) and stimulates the production of the satiety hormones (PYY and GLP-1)

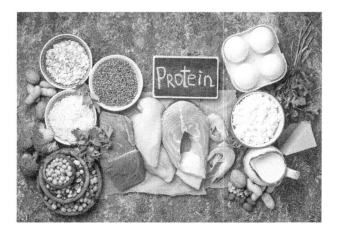

When you eat protein, it's transformed into amino acids, which help your body with various processes such as building muscle and regulating immune function.

However, many studies have established that red meat, processed meats, and highly processed meats promote and aggravate inflammation.

On the adapted whole foods diet, animal protein is consumed very moderately following the degree of food processing. You have to select animal sources of protein from the NOVA food group 1 (unprocessed or minimally processed), which include:

- poultry meat (fresh, chilled, or frozen), whole, steaks, fillets, and other cuts
- fish (fresh, chilled, or frozen), whole, steaks, fillets, and other cuts

You have also to choose vegetable sources of protein from the NOVA food group 1 (unprocessed or minimally processed), which include:

- lentils
- chickpeas
- green peas
- nuts
- seeds
- quinoa
- wild rice
- broccoli
- spinach
- asparagus
- artichokes
- sweet potatoes
- Brussels sprouts

Guidelines for individualized protein intake

The RDA (international Recommended Dietary Allowance) for protein is 0.8 g per kg of body weight, regardless of age. This recommendation is derived as the minimum amount to maintain nitrogen balance; however, it is not optimized for women's needs or physical activity levels.

Based on a recent body of evidence, the protein recommended intake from all sources can be adjusted to 1.4-1.8 grams per kg of your body weight.

The Protein Quality

The optimal source of protein is based on the calculation of the PDCAA (Protein Digestibility Corrected Amino Acid) Score or the DIAA (Digestibility Indispensable Amino Acid) Score. Thus, animal-based foods were identified as a superior source of protein because they offer a complete composition of essential amino acids, with higher bioavailability and digestibility (>90%). Thus, you have to eat a combination of animal proteins and plant proteins, mainly in the NOVA group 1 of foods (unprocessed and minimally processed).

Collagen, an essential ingredient

The most abundant type of protein in your body is collagen. Ligaments, tendons, skin, hair, nails, discs, and bones are collagen. Collagen is rich in amino acids that play an essential role in the building of joint cartilage. It also plays an important role in strengthening and rebuilding the lining of our digestive tract, thus healing gut inflammation and subsequently improving the immune system and helping modulate inflammation.

During the normal aging process, your body begins to experience a decline in the synthesis of collagen proteins. According to studies, this decline in collagen production starts around 30, at a rate of 1% per year. At the age of fifty, the rate jump to up to 3%, causing health issues::

- Muscle stiffness
- Aging joint
- Wrinkles and fine lines

- Lack of tone
- Aging skin
- Healing of wounds slower
- Frequent fatigue.

Consuming more collagen will boost your body's collagen protection. So it is recommended that your daily intake of collagen represent up to 25% of protein.

The beneficial effects include:

• Decreased gut inflammation.

• Improved intestinal health.

• Less articular pain.

• Less hair loss.

• Better skin.

• Increased muscle mass.

Foods rich in collagen

Here are some of the best collagen-rich foods you can add to your diet:

Bone broth

Made by simmering bones, tendons, ligaments, and skin of beef, bone broth is an excellent source of collagen and several essential amino acids. Bone broth is also available in powder, bar, or even capsules, so you can add it to your diet as a supplement.

Spirulina

This seaweed is an excellent source of plant-based amino acids, which are a key component of collagen. Spirulina can be found in dried form at most health food stores.

Codfish

Codfish, like most other types of white fish, is a good source of collagen in addition to selenium, vitamin B6 and phosphorus.

Eggs

Eggs are a good source of collagen, including glycine and proline.

---

3. Fats

After carbohydrates and proteins, it is essential to optimize the choice of your dietary fat.

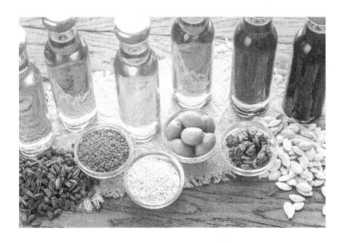

What is fat, and why it is essential for your health?

Dietary fats are found in both animals and vegetables and are essential for your living since they provide your body energy and support cell growth.

Fats also provide some valuable benefits and play essential roles, including:

- helping your body absorb some nutrients such as vitamins A, D, E, and K.

- helping your body produce the necessary hormones.
- regulating inflammation and immunity issues.
- maintaining the health of your cells (skin, hair cells)

How many different fats are there?

There are four major fats in food, based on their chemical structures and physical properties:

- Saturated fat (bad fat; reduce your intake of saturated fat): is a kind of fat in which the fatty acid chain of carbon atoms holds as many hydrogen atoms as possible (saturated with hydrogens). This form of saturated fat is associated with various adverse health effects, including aggravation of inflammation.
- Trans fat (very bad fat; to exclude completely): (trans-unsaturated fatty acids or trans fatty acids) are a form of unsaturated fat associated with various adverse health effects and known to worsen inflammation.
- Monounsaturated fats (healthy fat): are a type of unsaturated fat but have only one double bond. These fats are associated with positive health effects and may replace bad fats. Monounsaturated fats are found in olive oil, avocados, and some nuts
- Polyunsaturated fat (healthy fat): The two major classes of polyunsaturated fats are omega-3 and omega-6 fatty acids. However, many studies have shown that omega-3 and omega-6 have different inflammatory properties. Omega-3 fatty acids have powerful anti-inflammatory effects, while omega-6 tend to promote inflammation.

What is cholesterol?

Cholesterol is a waxy, fat-like substance found in all the cells in your body. Plus, your body needs some cholesterol to produce steroid hormones, vitamin D, and bile acid that helps you digest fats.

Contrary to popular belief, your body makes all the cholesterol it needs in the liver. Cholesterol is supplied in small quantities (less than 15%) by plant and animals foods.

More than 85% of the cholesterol in your bloodstream comes from your liver rather than from the food you eat. Dietary cholesterol has little impact on raising blood cholesterol levels, which is valuable information from a diet perspective.

A recent and growing body of evidence has pointed to inflammation as the most important cause of cardiovascular diseases rather than cholesterol. While a high cholesterol level in the blood can be dangerous, maintaining the right balance of cholesterol is essential for your health.

What types of fat should you eat?

Eating an adapted whole foods diet implies selecting fats found naturally in food and not being processed. You have then to choose fat-rich foods belonging to the NOVA group 1 of foods (unprocessed and minimally processed foods).

Examples of healthy sources of fat include:

- butter and ghee (clarified butter)
- cheese
- avocado (the fruit or avocado oil)
- cacao butter and powder
- sardines, anchovies
- salmon
- olives and olive oil
- macadamias and macadamia oil
- almonds and almonds oil
- Brazil nuts and Brazil nuts oil
- hazelnuts and hazelnuts oil
- pecan and pecan oil

What Are Fatty Acids?

Fatty acids are a form of hydrocarbon chains with carboxyl at one end and methyl at the other. The bioloGical activity of fatty acids is determined by the length of their carbon chain and their double bonds' number and position.

While saturated fatty acids do not contain double bonds within the acyl chain, unsaturated fatty acids include at least one double bond.

When two or more double bonds are present in their chain, unsaturated fatty acids are referred to as Dietary polyunsaturated fatty acids (PUFAs) and have been associated with cholesterol-lowering properties. The two families of PUFA are omega-3 and omega-6.

What Are Omega-3 Fatty Acids?

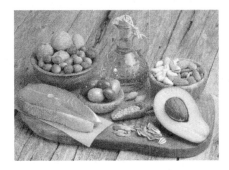

Omega-3 fatty acids are a type of polyunsaturated fats that the body can't produce. Omega-3 fatty acids are essential fats, so you have to get them from your diet.

There are various types of omega-3 fats, which differ by their chemical structure. The three most common types of omega-3 are:

- Eicosapentaenoic acid (EPA)
- Docosahexaenoic acid (DHA)
- Alpha-linolenic acid (ALA)

What Are Omega-6 Fatty Acids?

Like omega-3, omega-6 fatty acids are polyunsaturated fatty acids. omega-6 fatty acids are abundant and account for most polyunsaturated fatty acids in the food supply.

Following different recommendations and guidelines, we recommend a ratio of 4/1 omega-6 to omega-3 or less, which means that for 400 milligrams of omega-6, you have to consume 100 milligrams of omega-3. However, the Western diet has a very high ratio between 10/1 and 50/1.

Why and how is the excess of omega-6 harmful?

A high amount of omega-6 polyunsaturated fatty acids associated with a very high ratio of omega-6/omega-3 is a constant in most Western diets, including the keto diet. That increases the pathogenesis of several diseases, such as cancer, cardiovascular disease, autoimmune and inflammatory diseases. Conversely, high levels of omega-3 associated with a low ratio of omega-6/omega-3 induce health benefits. For example, a ratio omega-6/omega-3 of 4/1 was correlated to a 70% reduction in mortality.

This explains why the notion of the omega-6 / omega-3 ratio is essential in weight loss and health management.

Consuming fatty fish twice a week, eating whole foods, choosing dairy products and meat from grass-fed animals can help you improve your omega-6:omega-3 ratio.

10

FOOD PROCESSING CLASSIFICATION: OVERVIEW

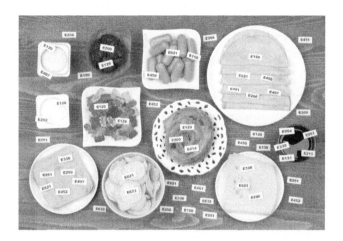

Food processing has been practiced for centuries in form of cooking, dehydrating, fermenting, ultraviolet radiation, and salt preservation. However, modern food processing methods are more sophisticated and complex, and alter considerably foods, by adding many ingredients including trans fats, high-fructose corn syrup, salts, artificial sweeteners, flavors, colors, and other chemical additives. The U.S. Department of Agriculture (USDA) defines processed food as one that has undergone any procedure that alters it from its natural state.

Thus, the current definition of processed food is broad, making a diet —like the whole foods diet— that excludes all processed food very hard and challenging to follow.

Therefore, we have to distinguish between healthy processed foods to include in the whole foods diet and those to exclude because considered unhealthy and pro-inflammatory.

Because of the huge heterogeneity among industrially processed foods, researchers have developed frameworks to classify foods based on the category or complexity of processing operations, ranging from minimally to highly processed. The NOVA classification system groups all foods based on the nature, complexity, and outcomes of the industrial processes they undergo. The NOVA classification system is recognized as a legitimate system to classify foods according to their degree of processing by the World Health Organisation (WHO), and the Food and Agriculture Organization (FAO).

NOVA classifies foods and food products into four distinct groups.

- group 1 of the NOVA classification: Unprocessed, natural, or minimally processed foods
- group 2 of the NOVA classification: Processed culinary ingredients
- group 3 of the NOVA classification: Processed foods
- group 4 of the NOVA classification: Ultra-processed foods

However, it can be sometimes challenging to distinguish food that has been minimally processed, processed or highly processed. For example:

1. Plain yogurt belongs to group 1 (minimally processed), but adding food additives such as artificial sweeteners, stabilizers, or preservatives made it ultra-processed (group 4).
2. Freshly made pizzas made from wheat flour, water, salt and yeast, garlic clove, onions, green peppers, black olives,

organic mozzarella cheese, raw parmesan cheese, red pepper, belongs to group 3 (processed), but adding food additives such as artificial sweeteners, stabilizers, or changing mozzarella cheese with a non-dairy cheese analog for pizza made it ultra-processed (group 4).

Group 1: Unprocessed or minimally processed foods

Unprocessed or whole foods are obtained directly from plants or animals and include the natural edible food parts of plants and animals.

Minimally processed foods are obtained from unprocessed or natural foods after minimal industrial processing that aims to enhance the edibility and digestibility of food or to increase its shelf life and storability without changing its nutritional content. Food undergoes minor transformations such as removal of non-edible or unwanted parts, crushing, drying, fractioning, grinding, roasting, refrigeration, freezing, vacuum packaging, boiling, pasteurization, non-alcoholic fermentation. The most commonly eaten unprocessed or minimally processed foods are:

- Natural, packaged, cut, chilled, or frozen vegetables
- Natural, packaged, cut, chilled, or frozen fruits
- Natural, packaged, cut, chilled, or frozen salads
- nuts, and other seeds without sugar or salt
- bulk or packaged grains such as wholegrain, brown, parboiled rice, or corn kernel
- fresh and/or dried herbs and spices (e.g., basil, dill, oregano, pepper, rosemary, thyme, cinnamon, mint, parsley)
- garlic powder
- fresh or pasteurized fruit juices with no added sugar or other ingredients

- fresh or pasteurized vegetable juices with no added sugar or other ingredients
- fresh and dried mushrooms
- cereal grains (e.g. wheat, barley, rye, oats, and sorghum)
- chickpeas, lentils, beans, black beans, peas, chicken beans, and other legumes
- flours made from maize, wheat, corn, or oats, including flours fortified with iron, folic acid, vitamin B (thiamin and niacin)
- flakes, and grits made from maize, wheat, corn, or oats, including flours fortified with iron, folic acid, vitamin B (thiamin and niacin)
- meat (fresh, chilled, or frozen), whole, steaks, fillets, and other cuts
- poultry meat (fresh, chilled, or frozen), whole, steaks, fillets, and other cuts
- fish (fresh, chilled, or frozen), whole, fillets, steaks, and other cuts
- fresh and/or dried pasta, couscous, and polenta made from water and the flours/grits/flakes described above
- fresh or pasteurized milk
- yogurt unsweetened without added sugar, flavor, or additives
- eggs
- tea
- herbal infusions
- coffee
- dried fruits
- water (tap, spring, and mineral)

Group 2: Processed Culinary Ingredients

The next category of processed foods includes products extracted from unprocessed, minimally processed foods, or directly from nature by pressing, grinding, crushing, milling, drying, or refining.

This group of food referred to as processed culinary ingredients is rather considered as ingredients for cooking various, delicious, and nutritious meals or dishes at home and elsewhere. They are rarely consumed by themselves but used in combination with foods.

The most commonly used processed culinary ingredients foods are:

- oils made from seeds, including sunflower oil, soybean oil, corn oil, cottonseed oil, rapeseed oil, canola oil, grapeseed oil, safflower oil
- oils made from nuts, including almond oil, hazelnut oil, Brazil nut oil, Walnut oil, Macadamia nut oil, and pecan oil.
- oils made from fruits, including olive oil, avocado oil, peach oil, apricot oil, coconut oil
- vegetable oils with added anti-oxidants
- butter
- salted butter
- sugar (white, brown, and other types) obtained from cane or beet
- molasses obtained from cane or beet
- honey (natural)
- lard
- coconut fat
- maple syrup
- cane syrup
- Agave syrup
- salt (refined or raw, mined or from seawater)
- table salt with added drying agents
- potato starch
- corn starch

- starches extracted from other plants
- balsamic vinegar
- Cane vinegar
- Coconut vinegar
- Malt vinegar
- any combination of two items of the NOVA group 2 "processed culinary ingredients"
- any item of the NOVA group 2 "processed culinary ingredients" with added vitamins or minerals, such as iodized salt

Group 3: Processed Foods

Processed foods are prepared by adding salt, oil, fat, sugar, or other ingredients from group 2 to group 1 food. The transformation processes include preservation, cooking, fermentation. These foods usually are made from at least two or three ingredients and can be eaten without further preparation. This group of food includes cheeses, smoked and cured meats, freshly-made bread, salted and sugared nuts, bacon, tinned fruit in syrup, cider, beer, and wine.

Processed foods usually keep an equivalent nutritional value and most nutrients and constituents of the original food. However, when excessive sugar, salt, or saturated oil are added, foods of group 3 become nutritionally unbalanced and may aggravate inflammation.

The most commonly eaten processed foods are::

- legumes canned or bottled preserved in salt (brine) or vinegar, or by pickling
- vegetables canned or bottled preserved in salt (brine) or vinegar, or by pickling
- fruit canned or bottled, packed in syrup
- fruits in sugar syrup (with or without added antioxidants)

- canned fish, such as sardine and tuna, with or without added preservatives
- fish (salted, dried, smoked)
- cured meat (salted, dried, smoked)
- tomato extract concentrates, or pastes, (with salt and/or sugar)
- beef jerky
- freshly-made cheeses
- freshly-made bread made of wheat flour, salt, yeast, and water
- bacon
- nuts (salted or sugared)
- seeds (salted or sugared)
- fermented alcoholic beverages such as alcoholic cider, beer, and wine
- fermented non-alcoholic beverages such as cider

Group 4: Ultra-processed foods

Also commonly referred to—as highly processed foods, Ultra-processed foods usually contain substances that you would never add when cooking homemade food. These are foods from group 3 that undergo "heavily" transformation to maintain or improve their taste, texture, safety, freshness, or appearance by the incorporation of substances:

- derived from foods—such as sugar, oils, fats, carbohydrates, and proteins,—or
- derived from food constituents—such as hydrogenated fats and modified starch—, or
- synthesized in laboratories—such as flavor enhancers, preservatives, antioxidants, colors, and other food additives—

Ultra-processed foods are defined as "formulations of several ingredients mostly of exclusive industrial use which, besides sugar, salt, oils, and fats, include food ingredients not used in culinary preparations, in particular, flavor enhancers, preservatives, colors, antioxidants, sweeteners, emulsifiers, and other additives used to provide sensory attributes of natural or minimally processed foods and their culinary preparations or to disguise undesirable sensory attributes of the final product such as odor, appearance, texture, flavor, and taste of foods"

The most commonly eaten ultra-processed foods are:

- Industrialized breads
- packaged breads
- Pre-prepared meals (packaged)
- Pre-prepared fish (packaged)
- Pre-prepared vegetables (packaged)
- pre-prepared pizza and pasta dishes
- pre-prepared pasta dishes
- pre-prepared poultry 'nuggets' and 'sticks'
- pre-prepared fish 'nuggets' and 'sticks'
- Breakfast cereals
- Sausages and other reconstituted meat products
- fatty packaged snacks
- sweet savory or salty packaged snacks
- savory or salty packaged snacks
- biscuits (cookies)
- chocolates
- candies
- gum and jelly products
- sweet fillings
- confectionery products in general
- pasties
- buns and cakes
- industrially-made chips (e.g. potato chips, banana chips, lentil chips)

- soft drinks
- fruit drinks
- fruit juices
- fast foods
- tortilla Chips
- chip Dips
- microwave Popcorn
- pretzels
- salty snacks in general
- ice creams
- frozen desserts
- pre-prepared burgers
- hot dogs
- sausages
- cola, soda, and other carbonated soft drinks
- animal products made from remnants
- energy and sports drinks
- packaged hamburger and hot dog buns
- instant soups
- instant noodles
- canned, packaged sauces
- canned, packaged, or powdered desserts
- canned, packaged, or powdered drink mixes
- canned, packaged, or powdered seasonings
- canned, packaged, powdered desserts, drink mixes, and seasonings
- flavored cheese crackers
- baked products made with ingredients other than those in group 2 (processed culinary ingredients) such as hydrogenated vegetable fat, emulsifiers, flavors, and other food additives.
- breakfast cereals and bars
- dairy drinks, including chocolate milk
- sweetened and/or flavored yogurts, including fruit yogurts
- infant formulas and drinks

- meal replacement shakes or powders
- sweetened juices made from concentrate
- pastries
- cakes and cake mixes
- margarine and spreads
- distilled beverages such as whisky, vodka, gin, rum, tequila.

Understanding the food nutrition label

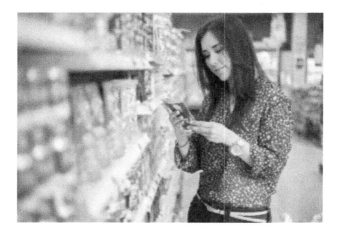

Food labeling regulation is complex, and food labels are filled with a multitude of numbers, percentages, and unusual ingredients making them difficult for consumers to understand. Products nutrition labels are often localized on the front, back, or side of the packaging. Food manufacturers must list on the product label all ingredients in the food to inform consumers what the food contains and to provide support in making healthier choices of processed foods.

Nutrition Facts label

A Nutrition Facts label breaks down the nutritional content of the food to help consumers to make healthier choices and compare between similar products. It includes

- the serving size,
- total fat,
- total carbohydrates,
- dietary fiber,
- protein,
- and vitamins per serving of the food

Example of using nutrition facts label:

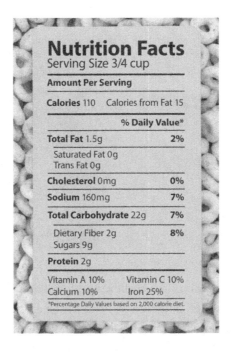

1. The first step is to check the **serving size.** All the values on this label are for a 3/4-cup serving.
2. **calorie** is an important value to many consumers. The label lists the calorie amount for one serving of food (110 calories for 3/4-cup in this example). So if you eat 1.5 cups, the total calorie is 220 calories.

3. **total fat** shows you types of fats in the food, including saturated fat, and trans fat. Avoid foods with trans fat. The total fat per 3/4-cup is 1.5 g
4. **total Carbohydrate** shows you types of carbohydrates in the food, including dietary fiber and sugar.
5. protein shows you the amount of protein in the food,
6. choose foods with lower calories, and that contain little amount of sugar, little amount of sodium, a high amount of fiber, more vitamins, and minerals.

Ingredients list

In addition to the nutrition label, food manufacturers are required to display ingredients label in their products. This is where consumers find all information about the constituents of the food, and can find if this product is suitable for them or not.

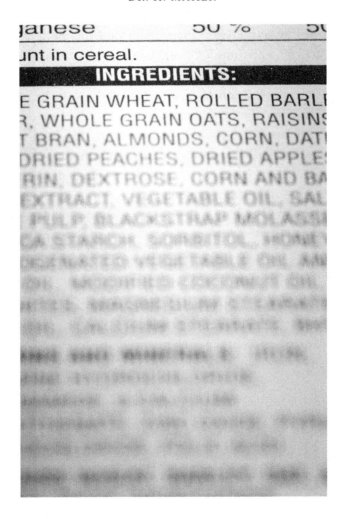

janese   5U %   5(

Jnt in cereal.

INGREDIENTS:

E GRAIN WHEAT, ROLLED BARLI
R, WHOLE GRAIN OATS, RAISIN!
T BRAN, ALMONDS, CORN, DAT!
DRIED PEACHES, DRIED APPLE!
RIN, DEXTROSE, CORN AND B/
EXTRACT, VEGETABLE OIL, SAL

Ingredients are listed in descending order of predominance— ingredients used in the greatest amount are listed first—. Food manufacturers are required to list food additives by their class name (e.g. acidity regulator, antioxidant, color, emulsifier, flavor enhancer, gelling agent, stabilizer, sweetener, thickener), followed by the name of the food additive or the food additive number.

11

MEAL PLANNING GUIDELINES

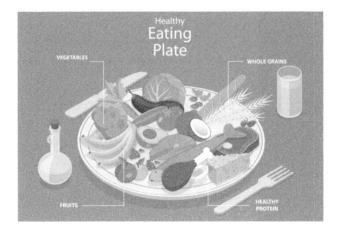

The glycemic index dietary guidelines ensure that recommendations for a healthy diet for diabetic people are met. Instead of giving strict recommendations, it gives options in each food group you can choose from. Each food has anti-inflammatory properties which significantly decrease the risk of diabetes complications and a low glycemic index.

All foods are assumed to be

- unprocessed or minimally processed (NOVA group I of Food (please refer to chapter 6 for more details),
- in nutrient-dense forms
- lean or low-fat
- prepared and cooked with minimal added sugars,
- prepared and cooked with minimal added salt (sodium)
- prepared and cooked with minimal refined carbohydrates, saturated fat, or trans fats.

The number of daily calories depends on your personal needs. You have to eat a balanced diet daily by following the general guidelines in this chapter and the amounts of food from each food group required to meet the glycemic index diet for diabetes goals. Recommended amounts of foods in each food group are given to allow you to design your weekly and monthly eating plan and may be adjusted to your own needs.

I- Vegetables

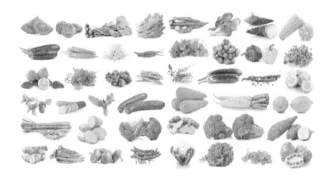

1.1 What is the portion size?

The typical serving size for vegetables and vegetable juices are equivalent to:

- 1 portion = 1 cup raw or salad vegetables
- 1 portion = 1/2 cup cooked vegetables
- 1 portion = 3/4 cup (6oz) vegetable juice homemade and unsweetened
- 1 portion = ½ cup of cooked beans, lentils, and peas

All vegetables are supposed to be low-glycemic-index and anti-inflammatory.

For moderate glycemic index vegetables divide the portion sizes by 2.

How Much a Day?

Total vegetable intake: up to 10 portions per day

- "Dark-Green Vegetables" group up to 2 servings
- "Red & Orange Vegetables" group up to 3 servings
- "Beans, Peas, Lentils" group up to 2 servings
- "Starchy Vegetables" group up to 1 serving
- "Other Vegetables" group up to 3 servings

For most people, following the glycemic index diet for diabetes will require an increase in total vegetable intake from all four vegetable subgroups ("Dark-Green Vegetables", "Red & Orange Vegetables", "Beans, Peas, Lentils", "Other Vegetables"). The consumption of "Starchy Vegetables" must be limited.

Strategies to increase total vegetable intake include

1. increasing the vegetable content of mixed dishes (more vegetables)
2. adding vegetables to breakfast
3. blending and consuming vegetables into smoothies
4. preparing sauces with vegetables
5. consuming regularly vegetable-based soups

1.2 Dark-Green Vegetables:

- **amaranth leaves** (all fresh, frozen, cooked, or raw)
- **arugula (rocket)** (all fresh, frozen, cooked, or raw)
- **bok choy (Chinese chard)** (all fresh, frozen, cooked, or raw)
- **dandelion greens** (all fresh, frozen, cooked, or raw)
- **kale** (all fresh, frozen, cooked, or raw)
- **mustard greens** (all fresh, frozen, cooked, or raw)
- **rapini (broccoli raab)** (all fresh, frozen, cooked, or raw)
- **swiss chard** (all fresh, frozen, cooked, or raw)
- **turnip greens** (all fresh, frozen, cooked, or raw)
- **broccoli** (all fresh, frozen, cooked, or raw)
- **chamnamul** (all fresh, frozen, cooked, or raw)
- **chard** (all fresh, frozen, cooked, or raw)
- **collards** (all fresh, frozen, cooked, or raw)
- **poke greens** (all fresh, frozen, cooked, or raw)
- **romaine lettuce** (all fresh, frozen, cooked, or raw)
- **spinach** (all fresh, frozen, cooked, or raw)
- **taro leaves** (all fresh, frozen, cooked, or raw)
- **watercress** (all fresh, frozen, cooked, or raw)

1.3 Red and Orange Vegetables

- **acorn squash** (all fresh, frozen, vegetables or juice, cooked or raw)
- **butternut squash** (all fresh, frozen, vegetables or juice, cooked or raw)
- **calabaza** (all fresh, frozen, vegetables or juice, cooked or raw)
- **carrots** (all fresh, frozen, vegetables or juice, cooked or raw)
- **red bell peppers** (all fresh, frozen, vegetables or juice, cooked or raw)

- **hubbard squash** (all fresh, frozen, vegetables or juice, cooked or raw)
- **orange bell peppers** (all fresh, frozen, vegetables or juice, cooked or raw)
- **sweet potatoes** (all fresh, frozen, vegetables or juice, cooked or raw)
- **tomatoes** (all fresh, frozen, vegetables or juice, cooked or raw)
- **pumpkin** (all fresh, frozen, vegetables or juice, cooked or raw)
- **winter squash** (all fresh, frozen, vegetables or juice, cooked or raw)

1.4 Beans, Peas, Lentils

- **beans** (all cooked from dry)
- **peas** (all cooked from dry)
- **chickpeas (Garbanzo Beans)** (all cooked from dry)
- **lentils** (all cooked from dry)
- **black beans** (all cooked from dry)
- **black-eyed peas** (all cooked from dry)
- **Bayo beans** (all cooked from dry)
- **cannellini beans** (all cooked from dry)
- **great northern beans** (all cooked from dry)
- **edamame** (all cooked from dry)
- **kidney beans** (all cooked from dry)
- **lentils** (all cooked from dry)
- **lima beans** (all cooked from dry)
- **mung beans** (all cooked from dry)
- **pigeon peas** (all cooked from dry)
- **pinto beans** (all cooked from dry)
- **split peas** (all cooked from dry)

1.5 Starchy Vegetables

- **breadfruit** (all fresh, or frozen)
- **burdock root** (all fresh, or frozen)
- **cassava** (all fresh, or frozen)
- **jicama** (all fresh, or frozen)
- **lotus root** (all fresh, or frozen)
- **plantains** (all fresh, or frozen)
- **salsify** (all fresh, or frozen)
- **taro root (dasheen or yautia)** (all fresh, or frozen)
- **water chestnuts** (all fresh, or frozen)
- **yam** (all fresh, or frozen)
- **yucca** (all fresh, or frozen)

1.6 Other Vegetables

- **asparagus** (all fresh, frozen, cooked, or raw)
- **avocado** (all fresh, frozen, cooked, or raw)
- **bamboo shoots** (all fresh, frozen, cooked, or raw)
- **beets** (all fresh, frozen, cooked, or raw)
- **bitter melon** (all fresh, frozen, cooked, or raw)
- **Brussels sprouts** (all fresh, frozen, cooked, or raw)
- **green cabbage** (all fresh, frozen, cooked, or raw)
- **savoy cabbage** (all fresh, frozen, cooked, or raw)
- **red cabbage** (all fresh, frozen, cooked, or raw)
- **cactus pads** (all fresh, frozen, cooked, or raw)
- **cauliflower** (all fresh, frozen, cooked, or raw)
- **celery** (all fresh, frozen, cooked, or raw)
- **chayote (mirliton)** (all fresh, frozen, cooked, or raw)
- **cucumber** (all fresh, frozen, cooked, or raw)
- **eggplant** (all fresh, frozen, cooked, or raw)

- **green beans** (all fresh, frozen, cooked, or raw)
- **kohlrabi** (all fresh, frozen, cooked, or raw)
- **luffa** (all fresh, frozen, cooked, or raw)
- **mushrooms** (all fresh, frozen, cooked, or raw)
- **okra** (all fresh, frozen, cooked, or raw)
- **onions** (all fresh, frozen, cooked, or raw)
- **radish** (all fresh, frozen, cooked, or raw)
- **rutabaga** (all fresh, frozen, cooked, or raw)
- **seaweed** (all fresh, frozen, cooked, or raw)
- **snow peas** (all fresh, frozen, cooked, or raw)
- **summer squash** (all fresh, frozen, cooked, or raw)
- **tomatillos** (all fresh, frozen, cooked, or raw)

2. Fruits

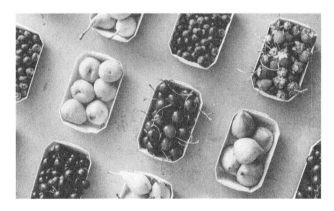

2.1 What is the portion size?

The typical portion sizes for low glycemic index fruits are equivalent to:

- 1 portion = 1 medium piece (120 grams)
- 1 portion = 1 cup (6 oz) of sliced fruits (120 grams)

- 1 portion = ⅓–½ cup of fruit juice
- 1 portion = 1-2 tablespoons of dried fruit

All fruits are supposed to be low-glycemic-index and anti-inflammatory.

For moderate glycemic index fruits divide the portion sizes by 2.

How Much a Day?

The current recommendation for people with diabetes is 2 to 4 portions of fruit per day. One portion contains 15 grams of carbohydrates if you use the carb counting method.

The fruit food group comprises whole fruits and fruit products (100% fruit juice). Whole fruits can be eaten in various forms, such as cut, cubed, sliced, or diced. At least 80% of the recommended amount of total fruit should come from whole fruit, rather than 100% juice. Juices should be without added sugars, food additives.

- **apples** (all fresh, frozen, dried fruits or 100% fruit juices)
- **Asian pears** (all fresh, frozen, dried fruits or 100% fruit juices)
- **bananas** (all fresh, frozen, dried fruits or 100% fruit juices)
- **blackberries** (all fresh, frozen, dried fruits or 100% fruit juices)
- **blueberries** (all fresh, frozen, dried fruits or 100% fruit juices)
- **currants** (all fresh, frozen, dried fruits or 100% fruit juices)
- **huckleberries** (all fresh, frozen, dried fruits or 100% fruit juices)
- **kiwifruit** (all fresh, frozen, dried fruits or 100% fruit juices)

- **mulberries** (all fresh, frozen, dried fruits or 100% fruit juices)
- **raspberries** (all fresh, frozen, dried fruits or 100% fruit juices)
- **strawberries** (all fresh, frozen, dried fruits or 100% fruit juices)
- **calamondin** (all fresh, frozen, dried fruits or 100% fruit juices)
- **grapefruit** (all fresh, frozen, dried fruits or 100% fruit juices)
- **lemons** (all fresh, frozen, dried fruits or 100% fruit juices)
- **limes** (all fresh, frozen, dried fruits or 100% fruit juices)
- **oranges** (all fresh, frozen, dried fruits or 100% fruit juices)
- **pomelos** (all fresh, frozen, dried fruits or 100% fruit juices)
- **cherries** (all fresh, frozen, dried fruits or 100% fruit juices)
- **dates** (all fresh, frozen, dried fruits or 100% fruit juices)
- **figs** (all fresh, frozen, dried fruits or 100% fruit juices)
- **grapes** (all fresh, frozen, dried fruits or 100% fruit juices)
- **guava** (all fresh, frozen, dried fruits or 100% fruit juices)
- **lychee** (all fresh, frozen, dried fruits or 100% fruit juices)
- **mangoes** (all fresh, frozen, dried fruits or 100% fruit juices)
- **nectarines** (all fresh, frozen, dried fruits or 100% fruit juices)
- **peaches** (all fresh, frozen, dried fruits or 100% fruit juices)
- **pears** (all fresh, frozen, dried fruits or 100% fruit juices)
- **plums** (all fresh, frozen, dried fruits or 100% fruit juices)
- **pomegranates** (all fresh, frozen, dried fruits or 100% fruit juices)
- **rhubarb** (all fresh, frozen, dried fruits or 100% fruit juices)
- **sapote** (all fresh, frozen, dried fruits or 100% fruit juices)
- **soursop** (all fresh, frozen, dried fruits or 100% fruit juices)

---

3. Grains

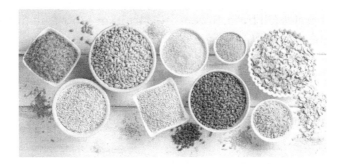

3.1 What is the portion size?

The typical portion sizes for low glycemic index cereals and grains are equivalent to:

- 1 portion = ⅓ cup breakfast cereal or muesli
- 1 portion = ½ cup of cooked cereal, or other cooked grain
- 1 portion = ⅓ cup of cooked rice (white rice excluded), and other small grains
- 1 portion = ½ cup of cold cereal

All breakfast cereals in this list below are low-glycemic-index and anti-inflammatory.

How Much a Day?

2-3 portions per day.

For moderate glycemic index cereals and grains divide the portion sizes by 2.

3.2 Whole grains

- **barley** (all whole-grain products or used as ingredients)
- **brown rice** (all whole-grain products or used as ingredients)
- **buckwheat** (all whole-grain products or used as ingredients)
- **bulgur** (all whole-grain products or used as ingredients)

- **millet** (all whole-grain products or used as ingredients)
- **oats (Avena sativa L.)** (all whole-grain products or used as ingredients)
- **quinoa** (all whole-grain products or used as ingredients)
- **dark rye** (all whole-grain products or used as ingredients)
- **whole-wheat bread** (all whole-grain products or used as ingredients)
- **whole-wheat chapati** (all whole-grain products or used as ingredients)
- **whole-grain cereals** (all whole-grain products or used as ingredients)
- **wild rice** (all whole-grain products or used as ingredients)

4. Dairy and Fortified Soy Alternatives

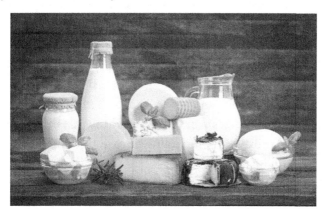

4.1 What is the portion size?

The typical portions sizes for dairy products are equivalent to:

- 1 portion = 1 medium glass of milk, soy beverage, or plain yogurt (200 ml)
- 1 portion = ⅓ cup of reduced or low-fat cheese (60 grams)

- 1 portion = 30g/1oz of hard cheese

All dairy and soy alternatives in this list are low-glycemic-index and anti-inflammatory.

People with celiac disease or lactose intolerance should consume dairy alternatives.

For moderate glycemic index dairy and soy alternatives divide the portion sizes by 2.

How Much a Day?

Up to 3 portions per day

- **buttermilk** (all fluid, evaporated milk, or dry including lactose-free and lactose-reduced products)
- **soy beverages** (all fluid, evaporated milk, or dry including lactose-free and lactose-reduced products)
- **soy milk** (all fluid, evaporated milk, or dry including lactose-free and lactose-reduced products)
- **yogurt** (without added sugar and food additives) (all fluid, evaporated milk, or dry including lactose-free and lactose-reduced products)
- **kefir** (without added sugar and food additives) (all fluid, evaporated milk, or dry including lactose-free and lactose-reduced products)
- **frozen yogurt** (without added sugar and food additives) (all fluid, evaporated milk, or dry including lactose-free and lactose-reduced products)
- **cheeses** (all fluid, evaporated milk, or dry including lactose-free and lactose-reduced products)

5. Protein Foods

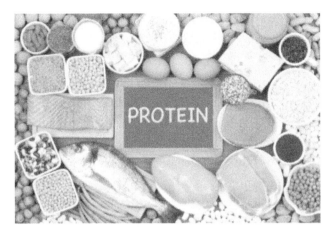

Eating an adequate amount of protein is extremely important for your health. Because Protein plays a crucial role in your body's vital processes and metabolisms, such as building and repairing tissues, building muscles, blood, hair, and skin, and producing hormones, enzymes, and other body chemicals.

Unlike carbohydrates and fat, your body does not store protein, and you need to eat the necessary amount to keep the right hormonal balance and fight unnecessary inflammation. Animal-based foods are identified as superior sources of protein because they offer a complete composition of essential amino acids, with higher bioavailability and digestibility (>90%). Therefore, the main principle to observe here when designing your meal program is to keep a weekly proteins intake equivalent to:

- 30 servings of animal proteins (mainly lean white meat and eggs)
- 10 servings of seafood
- 5 servings of nuts and seeds

5.1 Meats, Poultry, Eggs, Seafoods: what is the portion size?

The typical serving sizes for the "meats, poultry, eggs", "seafood", and "nuts, seeds, soy Products" groups are equivalent to:

- 1 portion = 3 to 4 ounces of cooked, baked, or broiled beef
- 1 portion = 3 to 4 ounces of cooked, baked, or broiled veal
- 1 portion = 3 to 4 ounces of cooked, baked, or broiled poultry
- 1 portion = 3 to 4 ounces of cooked or canned fish
- 1 portion = 3 to 4 ounces of seafood
- 1 portion = 2 medium eggs
- 1 portion = ⅓ cup of nuts (5 large or 10 small nuts)
- 1 portion = 2 tablespoons of nut butter
- 1 portion = 2 tablespoons of nut spread

5.2 Meats, Poultry, Eggs

Meats (lean or low-fats) include:

- beef, goat, lamb, pork (fat red meats must be limited due to their pro-inflammatory effects). You have to choose lean meats preferably grass-fed beef, lamb, or bison
- game meat (e.g., bison, moose, elk, deer)

Poultry (lean or low-fats) includes

- chicken
- turkey
- cornish hens
- duck
- game birds (e.g., ostrich, pheasant, and quail)
- goose.

Eggs include

- chicken eggs
- turkey eggs
- duck eggs and other birds' eggs

5.3 Seafood

Seafood include

- salmon
- sardine
- anchovy
- black sea bass
- catfish
- clams
- cod
- crab
- crawfish
- flounder
- haddock
- hake
- herring
- lobster
- mullet
- oyster
- perch
- pollock
- scallop
- shrimp
- sole
- squid
- tilapia

- freshwater trout
- tuna

5.4 Nuts, Seeds, Soy Products

Nuts (and nut butter) include

- almonds
- pecans
- Brazil nuts
- pistachios
- hazelnuts
- macadamias
- pine nuts
- walnuts
- cashew nuts

Seeds (and seed butter) include:

- pumpkin seeds
- psyllium seeds
- chia seeds.
- flax seeds
- sunflower seeds
- sesame seeds
- poppy seeds

12

LOW-GLYCEMIC EATING PRINCIPLES AND GUIDELINES

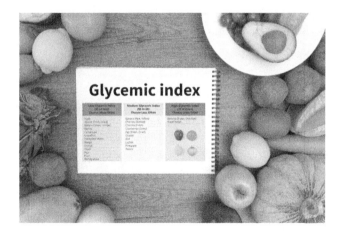

Dietary fiber in GI

Fiber plays a crucial role in weight loss
management, weight maintenance,
diabetes management and obesity control.

Fiber plays a crucial role
in weight loss
management because it
slows down the
absorption of sugars, and
digestion takes longer.

Tips

Raw fruit and vegetable are
lower in glycemic index than
juices, for example.

Facts

Dietary fiber comprises
many essential
molecules, including
cellulose, dextrins,
lignin, pectins, inulin,
chitins, waxes, beta-
glucans, and
oligosaccharides. the
higher dietary fibre
content frequently
associated with low-GI
foods may add to the
metabolic merits of a
low-GI diet.

Benefits

Eating a low glycemic diet
implies choosing foods
with high fiber content in
place of low-fiber foods,
provided their glycemic
index is low to moderate.

Unprocessed foods

Unprocessed foods are more complex to digest than processed foods, so they are generally low glycemic index.

Keep in mind that calories are not equal, and choose high-quality food by following the guidelines in this chapter.

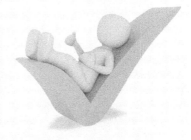

Tips

Eating a low glycemic diet implies choosing unprocessed foods in place of processed alternatives.

Facts

Studies show that the proportion of carbohydrates digested was significantly higher for processed foods than the unprocessed cooked foods, which produced a higher glycemic index.

Risks

processed foods are always suggested to be a great contributor to the obesity epidemic and rising prevalence of chronic diseases like inflammations, heart disease and type 2 diabetes

Fat in low GI diet

All kinds of fats lower the glycemic response of carbohydrates.

White bread with butter is harder to digest than white bread, so that you can reduce the glycemic index of foods using such a trick.

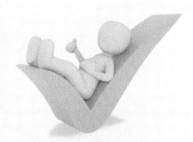

Tips

The first thing you have to do before starting the low glycemic diet is to figure out how much you need to lose.

Facts

When following the low glycemic index diet, it is essential to keep in mind that high-GI foods are not entirely banned. When eaten with fats, protein foods, or low-GI foods, or cooked firmly (like al dente for pasta) the overall GI value of the meal would be about low to medium.

Benefit

It is admitted that adding fat and protein to high-carbohydrate food content reduces glycemic responses by delaying gastric emptying and stimulating insulin secretion.

Cooking time in GI

Longer cooking time makes some foods easier to digest, increasing the blood sugar level.

Keep in mind that calories are not equal, and choose high-quality food by following the guidelines in this chapter.

Tips

When eating a low glycemic index diet, it is essential to remember that high-GI foods are not entirely banned.

Facts

When cooked al dente, pasta is more complex to digest than overcooked one. It has a lower glycemic index—reducing cooking time and eating foods while still firm means difficult digestion and smooth insulin release in the bloodstream.

Benefits

When eaten cooked firmly (like al dente for pasta), the new GI value of the meal would be about low to medium.

Protein in GI diet

Proteins slow the digestion of carbohydrates and lower the effects of high-glycemic-index food on your blood sugar.

Protein plays a crucial role in vital processes and metabolism of your body, such as building and repairing tissues, building muscles, blood, hair, and skin, and producing hormones, enzymes, and other body chemicals.

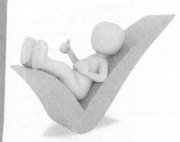

Tips

Eggs have a relatively low glycemic index and are perfect. So if you eat a boiled egg with your whole wheat bread or white bread toast, your meal will have a lower GI.

Benefits

You can eat high-glycemic index foods provided you combine them with low-glycemic index foods like eggs, olive oil, and butter.
The RDA (International Recommended Dietary Allowance) for protein is 0.8 g per kg of body weight, regardless of age.

Facts

The study "Egg ingestion in adults with type 2 diabetes" published in 2016 by a group of researchers showed that the daily inclusion of eggs in the habitual eating plan for 12 weeks reduced body weight, visceral fat rating, waist circumference, and percent body fat in adults with type 2 diabetes.

High GI Foods

Eating a low glycemic diet implies replacing high glycemic index foods with low glycemic index and moderate glycemic index alternatives.

When eating a low glycemic index diet, it is essential to remember that high-GI foods are not entirely banned.

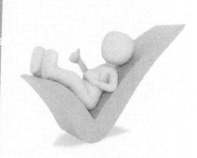

Tips

You can lower the negative impact of foods with a high glycemic index by combining them with low glycemic index foods.

Benefits

If you want to eat a white-bread bagel, for example, try adding a boiled egg or spreading it with a tablespoon of olive oil, butter, or peanut butter instead of jams or strawberry jelly.

Facts

Always remember that even small losses in weight can drive better health and sustainable weight loss.

Acidic drinks & foods

Foods that are considered acidic generally have a pH level of 4.6 or lower.

Keep in mind that although these foods have positive impact in GI, their initial acidity could worsen symptoms for those with upper gastrointestinal issues like an ulcer or reflux.

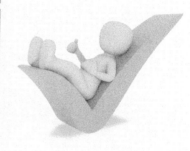

Tips

Adding Citrus fruits like lemons to meals with a high-glycemic index helps lower the meal's overall glycemic index.

Benefits

The addition of vinegar to starches-rich meals with a high-glycemic-index character reduces the meal's glycemic index and increases the post-meal satiety.

Facts

Many studies have reported the remarkable effect of acidic drinks and foods in reducing the glycemic response to carbohydrates-rich meals by 20 to 50%.

Omega-3 & GI diet

Omega-3 fatty acids are a type of
polyunsaturated fats classified as
"essential fats

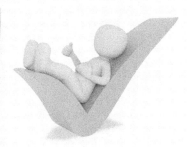

Keep in mind that calories
are not equal, and choose
high-quality food by
following the guidelines
in this chapter.

Tips

The best way to ensure optimal
omega-3 consumption is to eat
fatty fish at least twice per week.
However, if you don't eat fatty fish
or seafood, you may consider
taking a supplement.

Facts

The omega-3 fatty acids
have several potential
health benefits, including
supporting a weight loss
diet. Fish oil omega-3s
will help you lose inches
and shed body fat. The
USDA Food Guide Pyramid
recommends between 1
and 3 grams of omega-3
per day.

Benefits

Omega-3 is an essential fat
that you must integrate into
your low-glycemic diet.
They have significant
benefits for your heart,
brain, and metabolism.

Omega-6 in GI diet

Omega-6 fats from vegetable oils and other sources are good for the heart and body.

Good sources of omega-6 include : Safflower oil, sunflower oil, corn oil, soybean oil, sunflower seeds, walnuts, pumpkin seeds.

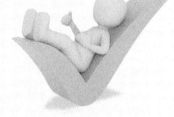

Tips

The first thing you have to do before starting the low glycemic diet is to figure out how much you need to lose.

Benefits

Following different recommendations and guidelines, we recommend a ratio of 4/1 omega-6 to omega-3 or less, which means that for 400 milligrams of omega-6, you have to consume 100 milligrams of omega-3.

Facts

Unlike saturated and trans fats, the polyunsaturated omega-3 and omega-6 fats and the monounsaturated fats are healthy, if consumed moderately.

Collagen & GI diet

The most abundant type of protein in your body is collagen.

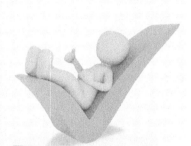

Keep in mind that calories are not equal, and choose high-quality food by following the guidelines in this chapter.

Tips

Ligaments, tendons, skin, hair, nails, discs, and bones are collagen. Eating collagen will positively impact them.

Benefits

Consuming more collagen will boost your body's collagen protection. So we recommend that your daily intake of collagen represents 25 to 35% of protein.

Facts

During the normal aging process, the body begins to experience a decline in the synthesis of collagen proteins around 30, at a rate of 1% per year. At the age of fifty, the rate jump to up to 3%, causing health issues: muscle stiffness, aching joints, wrinkles, and fine lines; lack of tone, sagging skin, healing of wounds slower, frequent fatigue.

PART II

3000+ BRAND-NAME AND GENERIC FOODS GI VALUES

13

BEEF, LAMP, VEAL, PORK & POULTRY

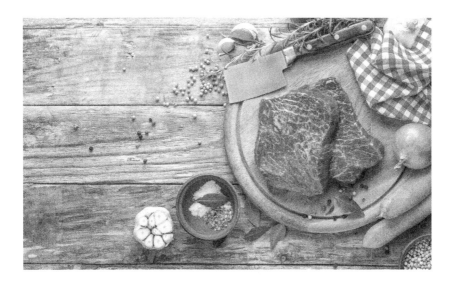

What is the serving size?

The typical serving sizes for low GI Meats are equivalent to:

- 3 to 4 ounces of cooked, baked, broiled, or canned beef
- 3 to 4 ounces of cooked, baked, broiled, or canned veal

- 3 to 4 ounces of cooked, baked, broiled, or canned poultry
- 3 to 4 ounces of cooked, baked, broiled, or canned fork
- 2 medium eggs

For moderate GI Beef, Lamb, Veal, Pork & Poultry products reduce the serving by 1/3

How Much a Day?

Up to 3 servings per day

Beef-Offal—Heart :Battered + fried ☛ GI = 95 (High)

Beef-Offal—Heart :braised ☛ GI = 50 (Low)

Beef-Offal—Heart :Breaded + fried ☛ GI = 95 (High)

Beef-Offal—Heart :Broiled and/or baked ☛ GI = 0 (Low)

Beef-Offal—Heart :Fried ☛ GI = 0 (Low)

Beef-Offal—Heart :Stewed ☛ GI = 0 (Low)

Beef-Offal—Heart ☛ GI = 0.0 (Low)

Beef—Bacon ☛ GI = 0.0 (Low)

Beef—blood sausage ☛ GI = 28 (Low)

Beef—Bologna ☛ GI = 0.0 (Low)

Beef—Bottom Round :Battered + fried ☛ GI = 95 (High)

Beef—Bottom Round :braised ☛ GI = 50 (Low)

Beef—Bottom Round :Breaded + fried ☛ GI = 95 (High)

Beef—Bottom Round :Broiled and/or baked ☛ GI = 0 (Low)

Beef—Bottom Round :Fried ☛ GI = 0 (Low)

🐄 Beef—Bottom Round :Roast ☛ GI = 0 (Low)

🐄 Beef—Bottom Round :Stewed ☛ GI = 0 (Low)

🐄 Beef—Bottom Round ☛ GI = 0.0 (Low)

🐄 Beef—Brain :Battered + fried ☛ GI = 95 (High)

🐄 Beef—Brain :braised ☛ GI = 50 (Low)

🐄 Beef—Brain :Breaded + fried ☛ GI = 95 (High)

🐄 Beef—Brain :Broiled and/or baked ☛ GI = 0 (Low)

🐄 Beef—Brain :Fried ☛ GI = 0 (Low)

🐄 Beef—Brain :Stewed ☛ GI = 0 (Low)

🐄 Beef—Brain ☛ GI = 0.0 (Low)

🐄 Beef—Brisket :Battered + fried ☛ GI = 95 (High)

🐄 Beef—Brisket :braised ☛ GI = 50 (Low)

🐄 Beef—Brisket :Breaded + fried ☛ GI = 95 (High)

🐄 Beef—Brisket :Broiled and/or baked ☛ GI = 0 (Low)

🐄 Beef—Brisket :Fried ☛ GI = 0 (Low)

🐄 Beef—Brisket :Roast ☛ GI = 0 (Low)

🐄 Beef—Brisket :Stewed ☛ GI = 0 (Low)

🐄 Beef—Brisket ☛ GI = 0.0 (Low)

🐄 Beef—Canned corned beef ☛ GI = 0.0 (Low)

🐄 Beef—Chorizo ☛ GI = 28 (Low)

🐄 Beef—Chuck Roast :Battered + fried ☛ GI = 95 (High)

🐄 Beef—Chuck Roast :braised ☛ GI = 50 (Low)

🐄 Beef—Chuck Roast :Breaded + fried ☛ GI = 95 (High)

Beef—Chuck Roast :Broiled and/or baked ☞ GI = 0 (Low)

Beef—Chuck Roast :Fried ☞ GI = 0 (Low)

Beef—Chuck Roast :Roast ☞ GI = 0 (Low)

Beef—Chuck Roast :Stewed ☞ GI = 0 (Low)

Beef—Chuck Roast ☞ GI = 0.0 (Low)

Beef—Chuck Steak Varieties Chart :Battered + fried ☞ GI = 95 (High)

Beef—Chuck Steak Varieties Chart :braised ☞ GI = 50 (Low)

Beef—Chuck Steak Varieties Chart :Breaded + fried ☞ GI = 95 (High)

Beef—Chuck Steak Varieties Chart :Broiled and/or baked ☞ GI = 0 (Low)

Beef—Chuck Steak Varieties Chart :Fried ☞ GI = 0 (Low)

Beef—Chuck Steak Varieties Chart :Roast ☞ GI = 0 (Low)

Beef—Chuck Steak Varieties Chart :Stewed ☞ GI = 0 (Low)

Beef—Chuck Steak Varieties Chart ☞ GI = 0.0 (Low)

Beef—Cured meats ☞ GI = 0.0 (Low)

Beef—Cuts of Steak :Battered + fried ☞ GI = 95 (High)

Beef—Cuts of Steak :braised ☞ GI = 50 (Low)

Beef—Cuts of Steak :Breaded + fried ☞ GI = 95 (High)

Beef—Cuts of Steak :Broiled and/or baked ☞ GI = 0 (Low)

Beef—Cuts of Steak :Fried ☞ GI = 0 (Low)

Beef—Cuts of Steak :Roast ☞ GI = 0 (Low)

Beef—Cuts of Steak :Stewed ☞ GI = 0 (Low)

🐄 Beef—Cuts of Steak ☞ GI = 0.0 (Low)

🐄 Beef—Delmonico Steak :Battered + fried ☞ GI = 95 (High)

🐄 Beef—Delmonico Steak :braised ☞ GI = 50 (Low)

🐄 Beef—Delmonico Steak :Breaded + fried ☞ GI = 95 (High)

🐄 Beef—Delmonico Steak :Broiled and/or baked ☞ GI = 0 (Low)

🐄 Beef—Delmonico Steak :Fried ☞ GI = 0 (Low)

🐄 Beef—Delmonico Steak :Roast ☞ GI = 0 (Low)

🐄 Beef—Delmonico Steak :Stewed ☞ GI = 0 (Low)

🐄 Beef—Delmonico Steak ☞ GI = 0.0 (Low)

🐄 Beef—Doner Kebab ☞ GI = 85 (High)

🐄 Beef—Frankfurter ☞ GI = 28 (Low)

🐄 Beef—Ground ☞ GI = 0.0 (Low)

🐄 Beef—Ham ☞ GI = 0.0 (Low)

🐄 Beef—Hamburger patty ☞ GI = 0.0 (Low)

🐄 Beef—Hanger Steak :Battered + fried ☞ GI = 95 (High)

🐄 Beef—Hanger Steak :braised ☞ GI = 50 (Low)

🐄 Beef—Hanger Steak :Breaded + fried ☞ GI = 95 (High)

🐄 Beef—Hanger Steak :Broiled and/or baked ☞ GI = 0 (Low)

🐄 Beef—Hanger Steak :Fried ☞ GI = 0 (Low)

🐄 Beef—Hanger Steak :Roast ☞ GI = 0 (Low)

🐄 Beef—Hanger Steak :Stewed ☞ GI = 0 (Low)

🐄 Beef—Hanger Steak ☞ GI = 0.0 (Low)

🐄 Beef—Kebab ☞ GI = 85 (High)

Beef—Kidney :Battered + fried ☛ GI = 95 (High)

Beef—Kidney :braised ☛ GI = 50 (Low)

Beef—Kidney :Breaded + fried ☛ GI = 95 (High)

Beef—Kidney :Broiled and/or baked ☛ GI = 0 (Low)

Beef—Kidney :Fried ☛ GI = 0 (Low)

Beef—Kidney :Stewed ☛ GI = 0 (Low)

Beef—Kidney ☛ GI = 0.0 (Low)

Beef—Liver :Battered + fried ☛ GI = 95 (High)

Beef—Liver :braised ☛ GI = 50 (Low)

Beef—Liver :Breaded + fried ☛ GI = 95 (High)

Beef—Liver :Broiled and/or baked ☛ GI = 0 (Low)

Beef—Liver :Fried ☛ GI = 0 (Low)

Beef—Liver :Stewed ☛ GI = 0 (Low)

Beef—Liver ☛ GI = 0.0 (Low)

Beef—Liver sausage ☛ GI = 0.0 (Low)

Beef—Liverwurst ☛ GI = 28 (Low)

Beef—Loin Steaks and/or Steak Types :Battered + fried ☛ GI = 95 (High)

Beef—Loin Steaks and/or Steak Types :braised ☛ GI = 50 (Low)

Beef—Loin Steaks and/or Steak Types :Breaded + fried ☛ GI = 95 (High)

Beef—Loin Steaks and/or Steak Types :Broiled and/or baked ☛ GI = 0 (Low)

Beef—Loin Steaks and/or Steak Types :Fried ☛ GI = 0 (Low)

🐄 Beef—Loin Steaks and/or Steak Types :Roast ☞ GI = 0 (Low)

🐄 Beef—Loin Steaks and/or Steak Types :Stewed ☞ GI = 0 (Low)

🐄 Beef—Loin Steaks and/or Steak Types ☞ GI = 0.0 (Low)

🐄 Beef—Low FODMAP Kebab ☞ GI = 85 (High)

🐄 Beef—luncheon meat ☞ GI = 28 (Low)

🐄 Beef—Meatball ☞ GI = 0.0 (Low)

🐄 Beef—Mettwurst ☞ GI = 0.0 (Low)

🐄 Beef—Mock Tender Petite Fillet :Battered + fried ☞ GI = 95 (High)

🐄 Beef—Mock Tender Petite Fillet :braised ☞ GI = 50 (Low)

🐄 Beef—Mock Tender Petite Fillet :Breaded + fried ☞ GI = 95 (High)

🐄 Beef—Mock Tender Petite Fillet :Broiled and/or baked ☞ GI = 0 (Low)

🐄 Beef—Mock Tender Petite Fillet :Fried ☞ GI = 0 (Low)

🐄 Beef—Mock Tender Petite Fillet :Roast ☞ GI = 0 (Low)

🐄 Beef—Mock Tender Petite Fillet :Stewed ☞ GI = 0 (Low)

🐄 Beef—Mock Tender Petite Fillet ☞ GI = 0.0 (Low)

🐄 Beef—Pastrami ☞ GI = 70 (High)

🐄 Beef—Pepperoni ☞ GI = 28 (Low)

🐄 Beef—Prime Rib :Battered + fried ☞ GI = 95 (High)

🐄 Beef—Prime Rib :braised ☞ GI = 50 (Low)

🐄 Beef—Prime Rib :Breaded + fried ☞ GI = 95 (High)

🐄 Beef—Prime Rib :Broiled and/or baked ☞ GI = 0 (Low)

🐄 Beef—Prime Rib :Fried ☞ GI = 0 (Low)

Beef—Prime Rib :Roast ☞ GI = 0 (Low)

Beef—Prime Rib :Stewed ☞ GI = 0 (Low)

Beef—Prime Rib ☞ GI = 0.0 (Low)

Beef—Rib Steak Cuts :Battered + fried ☞ GI = 95 (High)

Beef—Rib Steak Cuts :braised ☞ GI = 50 (Low)

Beef—Rib Steak Cuts :Breaded + fried ☞ GI = 95 (High)

Beef—Rib Steak Cuts :Broiled and/or baked ☞ GI = 0 (Low)

Beef—Rib Steak Cuts :Fried ☞ GI = 0 (Low)

Beef—Rib Steak Cuts :Roast ☞ GI = 0 (Low)

Beef—Rib Steak Cuts :Stewed ☞ GI = 0 (Low)

Beef—Rib Steak Cuts ☞ GI = 0.0 (Low)

Beef—Roasted ☞ GI = 0.0 (Low)

Beef—Round Steak Varieties :Battered + fried ☞ GI = 95 (High)

Beef—Round Steak Varieties :braised ☞ GI = 50 (Low)

Beef—Round Steak Varieties :Breaded + fried ☞ GI = 95 (High)

Beef—Round Steak Varieties :Broiled and/or baked ☞ GI = 0 (Low)

Beef—Round Steak Varieties :Fried ☞ GI = 0 (Low)

Beef—Round Steak Varieties :Roast ☞ GI = 0 (Low)

Beef—Round Steak Varieties :Stewed ☞ GI = 0 (Low)

Beef—Round Steak Varieties ☞ GI = 0.0 (Low)

Beef—Salami ☞ GI = 28 (Low)

Beef—Sausage ☞ GI = 0.0 (Low)

Beef—Sausage, Italian ☞ GI = 0.0 (Low)

🐄 Beef—Short Loin :Battered + fried ☛ GI = 95 (High)

🐄 Beef—Short Loin :braised ☛ GI = 50 (Low)

🐄 Beef—Short Loin :Breaded + fried ☛ GI = 95 (High)

🐄 Beef—Short Loin :Broiled and/or baked ☛ GI = 0 (Low)

🐄 Beef—Short Loin :Fried ☛ GI = 0 (Low)

🐄 Beef—Short Loin :Roast ☛ GI = 0 (Low)

🐄 Beef—Short Loin :Stewed ☛ GI = 0 (Low)

🐄 Beef—Short Loin ☛ GI = 0.0 (Low)

🐄 Beef—Short Ribs :Battered + fried ☛ GI = 95 (High)

🐄 Beef—Short Ribs :braised ☛ GI = 50 (Low)

🐄 Beef—Short Ribs :Breaded + fried ☛ GI = 95 (High)

🐄 Beef—Short Ribs :Broiled and/or baked ☛ GI = 0 (Low)

🐄 Beef—Short Ribs :Fried ☛ GI = 0 (Low)

🐄 Beef—Short Ribs :Roast ☛ GI = 0 (Low)

🐄 Beef—Short Ribs :Stewed ☛ GI = 0 (Low)

🐄 Beef—Short Ribs ☛ GI = 0.0 (Low)

🐄 Beef—T-Bone Steak :Battered + fried ☛ GI = 95 (High)

🐄 Beef—T-Bone Steak :braised ☛ GI = 50 (Low)

🐄 Beef—T-Bone Steak :Breaded + fried ☛ GI = 95 (High)

🐄 Beef—T-Bone Steak :Broiled and/or baked ☛ GI = 0 (Low)

🐄 Beef—T-Bone Steak :Fried ☛ GI = 0 (Low)

🐄 Beef—T-Bone Steak :Roast ☛ GI = 0 (Low)

🐄 Beef—T-Bone Steak :Stewed ☛ GI = 0 (Low)

🐄 Beef—T-Bone Steak ☞ GI = 0.0 (Low)

🐄 Beef—Tenderloin :Battered + fried ☞ GI = 95 (High)

🐄 Beef—Tenderloin :braised ☞ GI = 50 (Low)

🐄 Beef—Tenderloin :Breaded + fried ☞ GI = 95 (High)

🐄 Beef—Tenderloin :Broiled and/or baked ☞ GI = 0 (Low)

🐄 Beef—Tenderloin :Fried ☞ GI = 0 (Low)

🐄 Beef—Tenderloin :Roast ☞ GI = 0 (Low)

🐄 Beef—Tenderloin :Stewed ☞ GI = 0 (Low)

🐄 Beef—Tenderloin ☞ GI = 0.0 (Low)

🐄 Beef—Tongue :Battered + fried ☞ GI = 95 (High)

🐄 Beef—Tongue :braised ☞ GI = 50 (Low)

🐄 Beef—Tongue :Breaded + fried ☞ GI = 95 (High)

🐄 Beef—Tongue :Broiled and/or baked ☞ GI = 0 (Low)

🐄 Beef—Tongue :Fried ☞ GI = 0 (Low)

🐄 Beef—Tongue :Stewed ☞ GI = 0 (Low)

🐄 Beef—Tongue ☞ GI = 0.0 (Low)

🐄 Beef—Top Sirloin :Battered + fried ☞ GI = 95 (High)

🐄 Beef—Top Sirloin :braised ☞ GI = 50 (Low)

🐄 Beef—Top Sirloin :Breaded + fried ☞ GI = 95 (High)

🐄 Beef—Top Sirloin :Broiled and/or baked ☞ GI = 0 (Low)

🐄 Beef—Top Sirloin :Fried ☞ GI = 0 (Low)

🐄 Beef—Top Sirloin :Roast ☞ GI = 0 (Low)

🐄 Beef—Top Sirloin :Stewed ☞ GI = 0 (Low)

Beef—Top Sirloin ☛ GI = 0.0 (Low)

Beef—Tri-Tip :Battered + fried ☛ GI = 95 (High)

Beef—Tri-Tip :braised ☛ GI = 50 (Low)

Beef—Tri-Tip :Breaded + fried ☛ GI = 95 (High)

Beef—Tri-Tip :Broiled and/or baked ☛ GI = 0 (Low)

Beef—Tri-Tip :Fried ☛ GI = 0 (Low)

Beef—Tri-Tip :Stewed ☛ GI = 0 (Low)

Beef—Tri-Tip ☛ GI = 0.0 (Low)

Beef—Tripe :Battered + fried ☛ GI = 95 (High)

Beef—Tripe :braised ☛ GI = 50 (Low)

Beef—Tripe :Breaded + fried ☛ GI = 95 (High)

Beef—Tripe :Broiled and/or baked ☛ GI = 0 (Low)

Beef—Tripe :Fried ☛ GI = 0 (Low)

Beef—Tripe :Stewed ☛ GI = 0 (Low)

Beef—Tripe ☛ GI = 0.0 (Low)

Chicken—Backs and Necks :Battered + fried ☛ GI = 95 (High)

Chicken—Backs and Necks :braised ☛ GI = 50 (Low)

Chicken—Backs and Necks :Breaded + fried ☛ GI = 95 (High)

Chicken—Backs and Necks :Broiled and/or baked ☛ GI = 0 (Low)

Chicken—Backs and Necks :Fried ☛ GI = 0 (Low)

Chicken—Backs and Necks :Roast ☛ GI = 0 (Low)

Chicken—Backs and Necks :Stewed ☛ GI = 0 (Low)

Chicken—Backs and Necks ☛ GI = 0.0 (Low)

Chicken—Breast ☛ GI = 0.0 (Low)

Chicken—Breast Fillet Tenderloin :Battered + fried ☛ GI = 95 (High)

Chicken—Breast Fillet Tenderloin :braised ☛ GI = 50 (Low)

Chicken—Breast Fillet Tenderloin :Breaded + fried ☛ GI = 95 (High)

Chicken—Breast Fillet Tenderloin :Broiled and/or baked ☛ GI = 0 (Low)

Chicken—Breast Fillet Tenderloin :Fried ☛ GI = 0 (Low)

Chicken—Breast Fillet Tenderloin :Roast ☛ GI = 0 (Low)

Chicken—Breast Fillet Tenderloin :Stewed ☛ GI = 0 (Low)

Chicken—Breast Fillet Tenderloin ☛ GI = 0.0 (Low)

Chicken—Chorizo ☛ GI = 28 (Low)

Chicken—Cordon bleu (homemade) ☛ GI = 72 (High)

Chicken—Cordon bleu (industrially made) ☛ GI = 84 (High)

Chicken—Drumstick :Battered + fried ☛ GI = 95 (High)

Chicken—Drumstick :braised ☛ GI = 50 (Low)

Chicken—Drumstick :Breaded + fried ☛ GI = 95 (High)

Chicken—Drumstick :Broiled and/or baked ☛ GI = 0 (Low)

Chicken—Drumstick :Fried ☛ GI = 0 (Low)

Chicken—Drumstick :Roast ☛ GI = 0 (Low)

Chicken—Drumstick :Stewed ☛ GI = 0 (Low)

Chicken—Drumstick ☛ GI = 0.0 (Low)

Chicken—Leg :Battered + fried ☛ GI = 95 (High)

- Chicken—Leg :braised ☞ GI = 50 (Low)

- Chicken—Leg :Breaded + fried ☞ GI = 95 (High)

- Chicken—Leg :Broiled and/or baked ☞ GI = 0 (Low)

- Chicken—Leg :Fried ☞ GI = 0 (Low)

- Chicken—Leg :Roast ☞ GI = 0 (Low)

- Chicken—Leg :Stewed ☞ GI = 0 (Low)

- Chicken—Leg ☞ GI = 0.0 (Low)

- Chicken—Liverwurst ☞ GI = 28 (Low)

- Chicken—Luncheon meat ☞ GI = 0.0 (Low)

- Chicken—Nuggets ☞ GI = 46 (Low)

- Chicken—Pepperoni ☞ GI = 28 (Low)

- Chicken—Salami ☞ GI = 28 (Low)

- Chicken—Sausage ☞ GI = 28 (Low)

- Chicken—Tender :Battered + fried ☞ GI = 95 (High)

- Chicken—Tender :braised ☞ GI = 50 (Low)

- Chicken—Tender :Breaded + fried ☞ GI = 95 (High)

- Chicken—Tender :Broiled and/or baked ☞ GI = 0 (Low)

- Chicken—Tender :Fried ☞ GI = 0 (Low)

- Chicken—Tender :Roast ☞ GI = 0 (Low)

- Chicken—Tender :Stewed ☞ GI = 0 (Low)

- Chicken—Tender ☞ GI = 0.0 (Low)

- Chicken—Thigh :Battered + fried ☞ GI = 95 (High)

- Chicken—Thigh :braised ☞ GI = 50 (Low)

Chicken—Thigh :Breaded + fried ☛ GI = 95 (High)

Chicken—Thigh :Broiled and/or baked ☛ GI = 0 (Low)

Chicken—Thigh :Fried ☛ GI = 0 (Low)

Chicken—Thigh :Roast ☛ GI = 0 (Low)

Chicken—Thigh :Stewed ☛ GI = 0 (Low)

Chicken—Thigh ☛ GI = 0.0 (Low)

Chicken—Wing :Battered + fried ☛ GI = 95 (High)

Chicken—Wing :braised ☛ GI = 50 (Low)

Chicken—Wing :Breaded + fried ☛ GI = 95 (High)

Chicken—Wing :Broiled and/or baked ☛ GI = 0 (Low)

Chicken—Wing :Fried ☛ GI = 0 (Low)

Chicken—Wing :Roast ☛ GI = 0 (Low)

Chicken—Wing :Stewed ☛ GI = 0 (Low)

Chicken—Wing ☛ GI = 0.0 (Low)

Eggs—Free-Range ☛ GI = 0.0 (Low)

Eggs—Free-Run ☛ GI = 0.0 (Low)

Eggs—Organic ☛ GI = 0.0 (Low)

Eggs—Standard Brown ☛ GI = 0.0 (Low)

Lamb—Breast :Battered + fried ☛ GI = 95 (High)

Lamb—Breast :braised ☛ GI = 50 (Low)

Lamb—Breast :Breaded + fried ☛ GI = 95 (High)

Lamb—Breast :Broiled and/or baked ☛ GI = 0 (Low)

Lamb—Breast :Fried ☛ GI = 0 (Low)

🐑 Lamb—Breast :Roast ☞ GI = 0 (Low)

🐑 Lamb—Breast :Stewed ☞ GI = 0 (Low)

🐑 Lamb—Breast ☞ GI = 0.0 (Low)

🐑 Lamb—Cutlets :Battered + fried ☞ GI = 95 (High)

🐑 Lamb—Cutlets :braised ☞ GI = 50 (Low)

🐑 Lamb—Cutlets :Breaded + fried ☞ GI = 95 (High)

🐑 Lamb—Cutlets :Broiled and/or baked ☞ GI = 0 (Low)

🐑 Lamb—Cutlets :Fried ☞ GI = 0 (Low)

🐑 Lamb—Cutlets :Roast ☞ GI = 0 (Low)

🐑 Lamb—Cutlets :Stewed ☞ GI = 0 (Low)

🐑 Lamb—Cutlets ☞ GI = 0.0 (Low)

🐑 Lamb—Leg :Battered + fried ☞ GI = 95 (High)

🐑 Lamb—Leg :braised ☞ GI = 50 (Low)

🐑 Lamb—Leg :Breaded + fried ☞ GI = 95 (High)

🐑 Lamb—Leg :Broiled and/or baked ☞ GI = 0 (Low)

🐑 Lamb—Leg :Fried ☞ GI = 0 (Low)

🐑 Lamb—Leg :Roast ☞ GI = 0 (Low)

🐑 Lamb—Leg :Stewed ☞ GI = 0 (Low)

🐑 Lamb—Leg ☞ GI = 0.0 (Low)

🐑 Lamb—Loin :Battered + fried ☞ GI = 95 (High)

🐑 Lamb—Loin :braised ☞ GI = 50 (Low)

🐑 Lamb—Loin :Breaded + fried ☞ GI = 95 (High)

🐑 Lamb—Loin :Broiled and/or baked ☞ GI = 0 (Low)

🐑 Lamb—Loin :Fried ☞ GI = 0 (Low)

🐑 Lamb—Loin :Roast ☞ GI = 0 (Low)

🐑 Lamb—Loin :Stewed ☞ GI = 0 (Low)

🐑 Lamb—Loin ☞ GI = 0.0 (Low)

🐑 Lamb—Neck :Battered + fried ☞ GI = 95 (High)

🐑 Lamb—Neck :braised ☞ GI = 50 (Low)

🐑 Lamb—Neck :Breaded + fried ☞ GI = 95 (High)

🐑 Lamb—Neck :Broiled and/or baked ☞ GI = 0 (Low)

🐑 Lamb—Neck :Fried ☞ GI = 0 (Low)

🐑 Lamb—Neck :Roast ☞ GI = 0 (Low)

🐑 Lamb—Neck :Stewed ☞ GI = 0 (Low)

🐑 Lamb—Neck ☞ GI = 0.0 (Low)

🐑 Lamb—Rack :Battered + fried ☞ GI = 95 (High)

🐑 Lamb—Rack :braised ☞ GI = 50 (Low)

🐑 Lamb—Rack :Breaded + fried ☞ GI = 95 (High)

🐑 Lamb—Rack :Broiled and/or baked ☞ GI = 0 (Low)

🐑 Lamb—Rack :Fried ☞ GI = 0 (Low)

🐑 Lamb—Rack :Roast ☞ GI = 0 (Low)

🐑 Lamb—Rack :Stewed ☞ GI = 0 (Low)

🐑 Lamb—Rack ☞ GI = 0.0 (Low)

🐑 Lamb—Rump :Battered + fried ☞ GI = 95 (High)

🐑 Lamb—Rump :braised ☞ GI = 50 (Low)

🐑 Lamb—Rump :Breaded + fried ☞ GI = 95 (High)

Lamb—Rump :Broiled and/or baked ☞ GI = 0 (Low)

Lamb—Rump :Fried ☞ GI = 0 (Low)

Lamb—Rump :Roast ☞ GI = 0 (Low)

Lamb—Rump :Stewed ☞ GI = 0 (Low)

Lamb—Rump ☞ GI = 0.0 (Low)

Lamb—Shank :Battered + fried ☞ GI = 95 (High)

Lamb—Shank :braised ☞ GI = 50 (Low)

Lamb—Shank :Breaded + fried ☞ GI = 95 (High)

Lamb—Shank :Broiled and/or baked ☞ GI = 0 (Low)

Lamb—Shank :Fried ☞ GI = 0 (Low)

Lamb—Shank :Roast ☞ GI = 0 (Low)

Lamb—Shank :Stewed ☞ GI = 0 (Low)

Lamb—Shank ☞ GI = 0.0 (Low)

Lamb—Shoulder :Battered + fried ☞ GI = 95 (High)

Lamb—Shoulder :braised ☞ GI = 50 (Low)

Lamb—Shoulder :Breaded + fried ☞ GI = 95 (High)

Lamb—Shoulder :Broiled and/or baked ☞ GI = 0 (Low)

Lamb—Shoulder :Fried ☞ GI = 0 (Low)

Lamb—Shoulder :Roast ☞ GI = 0 (Low)

Lamb—Shoulder :Stewed ☞ GI = 0 (Low)

Lamb—Shoulder ☞ GI = 0.0 (Low)

Pork—back ribs :Battered + fried ☞ GI = 95 (High)

Pork—back ribs :braised ☞ GI = 50 (Low)

Pork—back ribs :Breaded + fried ☛ GI = 95 (High)

Pork—back ribs :Broiled and/or baked ☛ GI = 0 (Low)

Pork—back ribs :Fried ☛ GI = 0 (Low)

Pork—back ribs :Roast ☛ GI = 0 (Low)

Pork—back ribs :Stewed ☛ GI = 0 (Low)

Pork—back ribs ☛ GI = 0.0 (Low)

Pork—Belly :Battered + fried ☛ GI = 95 (High)

Pork—Belly :braised ☛ GI = 50 (Low)

Pork—Belly :Breaded + fried ☛ GI = 95 (High)

Pork—Belly :Broiled and/or baked ☛ GI = 0 (Low)

Pork—Belly :Fried ☛ GI = 0 (Low)

Pork—Belly :Roast ☛ GI = 0 (Low)

Pork—Belly :Stewed ☛ GI = 0 (Low)

Pork—Belly ☛ GI = 0.0 (Low)

Pork—Cutlets :Battered + fried ☛ GI = 95 (High)

Pork—Cutlets :braised ☛ GI = 50 (Low)

Pork—Cutlets :Breaded + fried ☛ GI = 95 (High)

Pork—Cutlets :Broiled and/or baked ☛ GI = 0 (Low)

Pork—Cutlets :Fried ☛ GI = 0 (Low)

Pork—Cutlets :Roast ☛ GI = 0 (Low)

Pork—Cutlets :Stewed ☛ GI = 0 (Low)

Pork—Cutlets ☛ GI = 0.0 (Low)

Pork—Garlic Sausages :Battered + fried ☛ GI = 95 (High)

🐷 Pork—Garlic Sausages :braised ☞ GI = 50 (Low)

🐷 Pork—Garlic Sausages :Breaded + fried ☞ GI = 95 (High)

🐷 Pork—Garlic Sausages :Broiled and/or baked ☞ GI = 0 (Low)

🐷 Pork—Garlic Sausages :Fried ☞ GI = 0 (Low)

🐷 Pork—Garlic Sausages :Roast ☞ GI = 0 (Low)

🐷 Pork—Garlic Sausages :Stewed ☞ GI = 0 (Low)

🐷 Pork—Garlic Sausages ☞ GI = 0.0 (Low)

🐷 Pork—Ham :Battered + fried ☞ GI = 95 (High)

🐷 Pork—Ham :braised ☞ GI = 50 (Low)

🐷 Pork—Ham :Breaded + fried ☞ GI = 95 (High)

🐷 Pork—Ham :Broiled and/or baked ☞ GI = 0 (Low)

🐷 Pork—Ham :Fried ☞ GI = 0 (Low)

🐷 Pork—Ham :Roast ☞ GI = 0 (Low)

🐷 Pork—Ham :Stewed ☞ GI = 0 (Low)

🐷 Pork—Ham ☞ GI = 0.0 (Low)

🐷 Pork—Loin :Battered + fried ☞ GI = 95 (High)

🐷 Pork—Loin :braised ☞ GI = 50 (Low)

🐷 Pork—Loin :Breaded + fried ☞ GI = 95 (High)

🐷 Pork—Loin :Broiled and/or baked ☞ GI = 0 (Low)

🐷 Pork—Loin :Fried ☞ GI = 0 (Low)

🐷 Pork—Loin :Roast ☞ GI = 0 (Low)

🐷 Pork—Loin :Stewed ☞ GI = 0 (Low)

🐷 Pork—Loin ☞ GI = 0.0 (Low)

- Pork—Rib chops :Battered + fried ☞ GI = 95 (High)

- Pork—Rib chops :braised ☞ GI = 50 (Low)

- Pork—Rib chops :Breaded + fried ☞ GI = 95 (High)

- Pork—Rib chops :Broiled and/or baked ☞ GI = 0 (Low)

- Pork—Rib chops :Fried ☞ GI = 0 (Low)

- Pork—Rib chops :Roast ☞ GI = 0 (Low)

- Pork—Rib chops :Stewed ☞ GI = 0 (Low)

- Pork—Rib chops ☞ GI = 0.0 (Low)

- Pork—Roasts :Battered + fried ☞ GI = 95 (High)

- Pork—Roasts :braised ☞ GI = 50 (Low)

- Pork—Roasts :Breaded + fried ☞ GI = 95 (High)

- Pork—Roasts :Broiled and/or baked ☞ GI = 0 (Low)

- Pork—Roasts :Fried ☞ GI = 0 (Low)

- Pork—Roasts :Roast ☞ GI = 0 (Low)

- Pork—Roasts :Stewed ☞ GI = 0 (Low)

- Pork—Roasts ☞ GI = 0.0 (Low)

- Pork—Sausages :Battered + fried ☞ GI = 95 (High)

- Pork—Sausages :braised ☞ GI = 50 (Low)

- Pork—Sausages :Breaded + fried ☞ GI = 95 (High)

- Pork—Sausages :Broiled and/or baked ☞ GI = 0 (Low)

- Pork—Sausages :Fried ☞ GI = 0 (Low)

- Pork—Sausages :Roast ☞ GI = 0 (Low)

- Pork—Sausages :Stewed ☞ GI = 0 (Low)

🐷 Pork—Sausages ☞ GI = 0.0 (Low)

🐷 Pork—Shoulder chops :Battered + fried ☞ GI = 95 (High)

🐷 Pork—Shoulder chops :braised ☞ GI = 50 (Low)

🐷 Pork—Shoulder chops :Breaded + fried ☞ GI = 95 (High)

🐷 Pork—Shoulder chops :Broiled and/or baked ☞ GI = 0 (Low)

🐷 Pork—Shoulder chops :Fried ☞ GI = 0 (Low)

🐷 Pork—Shoulder chops :Roast ☞ GI = 0 (Low)

🐷 Pork—Shoulder chops :Stewed ☞ GI = 0 (Low)

🐷 Pork—Shoulder chops ☞ GI = 0.0 (Low)

🐷 Pork—Sirloin chops :Battered + fried ☞ GI = 95 (High)

🐷 Pork—Sirloin chops :braised ☞ GI = 50 (Low)

🐷 Pork—Sirloin chops :Breaded + fried ☞ GI = 95 (High)

🐷 Pork—Sirloin chops :Broiled and/or baked ☞ GI = 0 (Low)

🐷 Pork—Sirloin chops :Fried ☞ GI = 0 (Low)

🐷 Pork—Sirloin chops :Roast ☞ GI = 0 (Low)

🐷 Pork—Sirloin chops :Stewed ☞ GI = 0 (Low)

🐷 Pork—Sirloin chops ☞ GI = 0.0 (Low)

🐷 Pork—spare ribs :Battered + fried ☞ GI = 95 (High)

🐷 Pork—spare ribs :braised ☞ GI = 50 (Low)

🐷 Pork—spare ribs :Breaded + fried ☞ GI = 95 (High)

🐷 Pork—spare ribs :Broiled and/or baked ☞ GI = 0 (Low)

🐷 Pork—spare ribs :Fried ☞ GI = 0 (Low)

🐷 Pork—spare ribs :Roast ☞ GI = 0 (Low)

🖐 Pork—spare ribs :Stewed ☞ GI = 0 (Low)

🖐 Pork—spare ribs ☞ GI = 0.0 (Low)

🖐 Turkey—Backs and Necks :Battered + fried ☞ GI = 95 (High)

🖐 Turkey—Backs and Necks :braised ☞ GI = 50 (Low)

🖐 Turkey—Backs and Necks :Breaded + fried ☞ GI = 95 (High)

🖐 Turkey—Backs and Necks :Broiled and/or baked ☞ GI = 0 (Low)

🖐 Turkey—Backs and Necks :Fried ☞ GI = 0 (Low)

🖐 Turkey—Backs and Necks :Roast ☞ GI = 0 (Low)

🖐 Turkey—Backs and Necks :Stewed ☞ GI = 0 (Low)

🖐 Turkey—Backs and Necks ☞ GI = 0.0 (Low)

🖐 Turkey—Breast :Battered + fried ☞ GI = 95 (High)

🖐 Turkey—Breast :braised ☞ GI = 50 (Low)

🖐 Turkey—Breast :Breaded + fried ☞ GI = 95 (High)

🖐 Turkey—Breast :Broiled and/or baked ☞ GI = 0 (Low)

🖐 Turkey—Breast :Fried ☞ GI = 0 (Low)

🖐 Turkey—Breast :Roast ☞ GI = 0 (Low)

🖐 Turkey—Breast :Stewed ☞ GI = 0 (Low)

🖐 Turkey—Breast ☞ GI = 0.0 (Low)

🖐 Turkey—Breast Fillet Tenderloin :Battered + fried ☞ GI = 95 (High)

🖐 Turkey—Breast Fillet Tenderloin :braised ☞ GI = 50 (Low)

🖐 Turkey—Breast Fillet Tenderloin :Breaded + fried ☞ GI = 95 (High)

Turkey—Breast Fillet Tenderloin :Broiled and/or baked ☞ GI = 0 (Low)

Turkey—Breast Fillet Tenderloin :Fried ☞ GI = 0 (Low)

Turkey—Breast Fillet Tenderloin :Roast ☞ GI = 0 (Low)

Turkey—Breast Fillet Tenderloin :Stewed ☞ GI = 0 (Low)

Turkey—Breast Fillet Tenderloin ☞ GI = 0.0 (Low)

Turkey—Chorizo ☞ GI = 28 (Low)

Turkey—Drumstick :Battered + fried ☞ GI = 95 (High)

Turkey—Drumstick :braised ☞ GI = 50 (Low)

Turkey—Drumstick :Breaded + fried ☞ GI = 95 (High)

Turkey—Drumstick :Broiled and/or baked ☞ GI = 0 (Low)

Turkey—Drumstick :Fried ☞ GI = 0 (Low)

Turkey—Drumstick :Roast ☞ GI = 0 (Low)

Turkey—Drumstick :Stewed ☞ GI = 0 (Low)

Turkey—Drumstick ☞ GI = 0.0 (Low)

Turkey—Leg :Battered + fried ☞ GI = 95 (High)

Turkey—Leg :braised ☞ GI = 50 (Low)

Turkey—Leg :Breaded + fried ☞ GI = 95 (High)

Turkey—Leg :Broiled and/or baked ☞ GI = 0 (Low)

Turkey—Leg :Fried ☞ GI = 0 (Low)

Turkey—Leg :Roast ☞ GI = 0 (Low)

Turkey—Leg :Stewed ☞ GI = 0 (Low)

Turkey—Leg ☞ GI = 0.0 (Low)

Turkey—Liverwurst ☞ GI = 28 (Low)

Turkey—Pastrami ☞ GI = 70 (High)

Turkey—Pepperoni ☞ GI = 28 (Low)

Turkey—Salami ☞ GI = 28 (Low)

Turkey—Sausage ☞ GI = 28 (Low)

Turkey—Tender :Battered + fried ☞ GI = 95 (High)

Turkey—Tender :braised ☞ GI = 50 (Low)

Turkey—Tender :Breaded + fried ☞ GI = 95 (High)

Turkey—Tender :Broiled and/or baked ☞ GI = 0 (Low)

Turkey—Tender :Fried ☞ GI = 0 (Low)

Turkey—Tender :Roast ☞ GI = 0 (Low)

Turkey—Tender :Stewed ☞ GI = 0 (Low)

Turkey—Tender ☞ GI = 0.0 (Low)

Turkey—Thigh :Battered + fried ☞ GI = 95 (High)

Turkey—Thigh :braised ☞ GI = 50 (Low)

Turkey—Thigh :Breaded + fried ☞ GI = 95 (High)

Turkey—Thigh :Broiled and/or baked ☞ GI = 0 (Low)

Turkey—Thigh :Fried ☞ GI = 0 (Low)

Turkey—Thigh :Roast ☞ GI = 0 (Low)

Turkey—Thigh :Stewed ☞ GI = 0 (Low)

Turkey—Thigh ☞ GI = 0.0 (Low)

Turkey—Wing :Battered + fried ☞ GI = 95 (High)

Turkey—Wing :braised ☞ GI = 50 (Low)

Turkey—Wing :Breaded + fried ☞ GI = 95 (High)

🦃 Turkey—Wing :Broiled and/or baked 🐄 GI = 0 (Low)

🦃 Turkey—Wing :Fried 🐄 GI = 0 (Low)

🦃 Turkey—Wing :Roast 🐄 GI = 0 (Low)

🦃 Turkey—Wing :Stewed 🐄 GI = 0 (Low)

🦃 Turkey—Wing 🐄 GI = 0.0 (Low)

🐄 Veal-Offal—Heart :Battered + fried 🐄 GI = 95 (High)

🐄 Veal-Offal—Heart :braised 🐄 GI = 50 (Low)

🐄 Veal-Offal—Heart :Breaded + fried 🐄 GI = 95 (High)

🐄 Veal-Offal—Heart :Broiled and/or baked 🐄 GI = 0 (Low)

🐄 Veal-Offal—Heart :Fried 🐄 GI = 0 (Low)

🐄 Veal-Offal—Heart 🐄 GI = 0.0 (Low)

🐄 Veal—Bottom Round :Battered + fried 🐄 GI = 95 (High)

🐄 Veal—Bottom Round :braised 🐄 GI = 50 (Low)

🐄 Veal—Bottom Round :Breaded + fried 🐄 GI = 95 (High)

🐄 Veal—Bottom Round :Broiled and/or baked 🐄 GI = 0 (Low)

🐄 Veal—Bottom Round :Fried 🐄 GI = 0 (Low)

🐄 Veal—Bottom Round :Roast 🐄 GI = 0 (Low)

🐄 Veal—Bottom Round :Stewed 🐄 GI = 0 (Low)

🐄 Veal—Bottom Round 🐄 GI = 0.0 (Low)

🐄 Veal—Brain :Battered + fried 🐄 GI = 95 (High)

🐄 Veal—Brain :braised 🐄 GI = 50 (Low)

🐄 Veal—Brain :Breaded + fried 🐄 GI = 95 (High)

🐄 Veal—Brain :Broiled and/or baked 🐄 GI = 0 (Low)

Veal—Brain :Fried 🖝 GI = 0 (Low)

Veal—Brain 🖝 GI = 0.0 (Low)

Veal—Brisket :Battered + fried 🖝 GI = 95 (High)

Veal—Brisket :braised 🖝 GI = 50 (Low)

Veal—Brisket :Breaded + fried 🖝 GI = 95 (High)

Veal—Brisket :Broiled and/or baked 🖝 GI = 0 (Low)

Veal—Brisket :Fried 🖝 GI = 0 (Low)

Veal—Brisket :Roast 🖝 GI = 0 (Low)

Veal—Brisket :Stewed 🖝 GI = 0 (Low)

Veal—Brisket 🖝 GI = 0.0 (Low)

Veal—Chuck Roast :Battered + fried 🖝 GI = 95 (High)

Veal—Chuck Roast :braised 🖝 GI = 50 (Low)

Veal—Chuck Roast :Breaded + fried 🖝 GI = 95 (High)

Veal—Chuck Roast :Broiled and/or baked 🖝 GI = 0 (Low)

Veal—Chuck Roast :Fried 🖝 GI = 0 (Low)

Veal—Chuck Roast :Roast 🖝 GI = 0 (Low)

Veal—Chuck Roast :Stewed 🖝 GI = 0 (Low)

Veal—Chuck Roast 🖝 GI = 0.0 (Low)

Veal—Chuck Steak Varieties Chart :Battered + fried 🖝 GI = 95 (High)

Veal—Chuck Steak Varieties Chart :braised 🖝 GI = 50 (Low)

Veal—Chuck Steak Varieties Chart :Breaded + fried 🖝 GI = 95 (High)

Veal—Chuck Steak Varieties Chart :Broiled and/or baked 🖝 GI =

0 (Low)

🐾 Veal—Chuck Steak Varieties Chart :Fried ☛ GI = 0 (Low)

🐾 Veal—Chuck Steak Varieties Chart :Roast ☛ GI = 0 (Low)

🐾 Veal—Chuck Steak Varieties Chart :Stewed ☛ GI = 0 (Low)

🐾 Veal—Chuck Steak Varieties Chart ☛ GI = 0.0 (Low)

🐾 Veal—Cuts of Steak :Battered + fried ☛ GI = 95 (High)

🐾 Veal—Cuts of Steak :braised ☛ GI = 50 (Low)

🐾 Veal—Cuts of Steak :Breaded + fried ☛ GI = 95 (High)

🐾 Veal—Cuts of Steak :Broiled and/or baked ☛ GI = 0 (Low)

🐾 Veal—Cuts of Steak :Fried ☛ GI = 0 (Low)

🐾 Veal—Cuts of Steak :Roast ☛ GI = 0 (Low)

🐾 Veal—Cuts of Steak :Stewed ☛ GI = 0 (Low)

🐾 Veal—Cuts of Steak ☛ GI = 0.0 (Low)

🐾 Veal—Delmonico Steak :Battered + fried ☛ GI = 95 (High)

🐾 Veal—Delmonico Steak :braised ☛ GI = 50 (Low)

🐾 Veal—Delmonico Steak :Breaded + fried ☛ GI = 95 (High)

🐾 Veal—Delmonico Steak :Broiled and/or baked ☛ GI = 0 (Low)

🐾 Veal—Delmonico Steak :Fried ☛ GI = 0 (Low)

🐾 Veal—Delmonico Steak :Roast ☛ GI = 0 (Low)

🐾 Veal—Delmonico Steak :Stewed ☛ GI = 0 (Low)

🐾 Veal—Delmonico Steak ☛ GI = 0.0 (Low)

🐾 Veal—Hanger Steak :Battered + fried ☛ GI = 95 (High)

🐾 Veal—Hanger Steak :braised ☛ GI = 50 (Low)

🐄 Veal—Hanger Steak :Breaded + fried ☞ GI = 95 (High)

🐄 Veal—Hanger Steak :Broiled and/or baked ☞ GI = o (Low)

🐄 Veal—Hanger Steak :Fried ☞ GI = o (Low)

🐄 Veal—Hanger Steak :Roast ☞ GI = o (Low)

🐄 Veal—Hanger Steak :Stewed ☞ GI = o (Low)

🐄 Veal—Hanger Steak ☞ GI = 0.0 (Low)

🐄 Veal—Kidney :Battered + fried ☞ GI = 95 (High)

🐄 Veal—Kidney :braised ☞ GI = 50 (Low)

🐄 Veal—Kidney :Breaded + fried ☞ GI = 95 (High)

🐄 Veal—Kidney :Broiled and/or baked ☞ GI = o (Low)

🐄 Veal—Kidney :Fried ☞ GI = o (Low)

🐄 Veal—Kidney ☞ GI = 0.0 (Low)

🐄 Veal—Liver :Battered + fried ☞ GI = 95 (High)

🐄 Veal—Liver :braised ☞ GI = 50 (Low)

🐄 Veal—Liver :Breaded + fried ☞ GI = 95 (High)

🐄 Veal—Liver :Broiled and/or baked ☞ GI = o (Low)

🐄 Veal—Liver :Fried ☞ GI = o (Low)

🐄 Veal—Liver ☞ GI = 0.0 (Low)

🐄 Veal—Loin Steaks and/or Steak Types :Battered + fried ☞ GI = 95 (High)

🐄 Veal—Loin Steaks and/or Steak Types :braised ☞ GI = 50 (Low)

🐄 Veal—Loin Steaks and/or Steak Types :Breaded + fried ☞ GI = 95 (High)

🐖 Veal—Loin Steaks and/or Steak Types :Broiled and/or baked 🐗 GI = 0 (Low)

🐖 Veal—Loin Steaks and/or Steak Types :Fried 🐗 GI = 0 (Low)

🐖 Veal—Loin Steaks and/or Steak Types :Roast 🐗 GI = 0 (Low)

🐖 Veal—Loin Steaks and/or Steak Types :Stewed 🐗 GI = 0 (Low)

🐖 Veal—Loin Steaks and/or Steak Types 🐗 GI = 0.0 (Low)

🐖 Veal—Mock Tender Petite Fillet :Battered + fried 🐗 GI = 95 (High)

🐖 Veal—Mock Tender Petite Fillet :braised 🐗 GI = 50 (Low)

🐖 Veal—Mock Tender Petite Fillet :Breaded + fried 🐗 GI = 95 (High)

🐖 Veal—Mock Tender Petite Fillet :Broiled and/or baked 🐗 GI = 0 (Low)

🐖 Veal—Mock Tender Petite Fillet :Fried 🐗 GI = 0 (Low)

🐖 Veal—Mock Tender Petite Fillet :Roast 🐗 GI = 0 (Low)

🐖 Veal—Mock Tender Petite Fillet :Stewed 🐗 GI = 0 (Low)

🐖 Veal—Mock Tender Petite Fillet 🐗 GI = 0.0 (Low)

🐖 Veal—Prime Rib :Battered + fried 🐗 GI = 95 (High)

🐖 Veal—Prime Rib :braised 🐗 GI = 50 (Low)

🐖 Veal—Prime Rib :Breaded + fried 🐗 GI = 95 (High)

🐖 Veal—Prime Rib :Broiled and/or baked 🐗 GI = 0 (Low)

🐖 Veal—Prime Rib :Fried 🐗 GI = 0 (Low)

🐖 Veal—Prime Rib :Roast 🐗 GI = 0 (Low)

🐖 Veal—Prime Rib :Stewed 🐗 GI = 0 (Low)

🐖 Veal—Prime Rib 🐗 GI = 0.0 (Low)

🐖 Veal—Rib Steak Cuts :Battered + fried 🐗 GI = 95 (High)

Veal—Rib Steak Cuts :braised ☞ GI = 50 (Low)

Veal—Rib Steak Cuts :Breaded + fried ☞ GI = 95 (High)

Veal—Rib Steak Cuts :Broiled and/or baked ☞ GI = 0 (Low)

Veal—Rib Steak Cuts :Fried ☞ GI = 0 (Low)

Veal—Rib Steak Cuts :Roast ☞ GI = 0 (Low)

Veal—Rib Steak Cuts :Stewed ☞ GI = 0 (Low)

Veal—Rib Steak Cuts ☞ GI = 0.0 (Low)

Veal—Round Steak Varieties :Battered + fried ☞ GI = 95 (High)

Veal—Round Steak Varieties :braised ☞ GI = 50 (Low)

Veal—Round Steak Varieties :Breaded + fried ☞ GI = 95 (High)

Veal—Round Steak Varieties :Broiled and/or baked ☞ GI = 0 (Low)

Veal—Round Steak Varieties :Fried ☞ GI = 0 (Low)

Veal—Round Steak Varieties :Roast ☞ GI = 0 (Low)

Veal—Round Steak Varieties :Stewed ☞ GI = 0 (Low)

Veal—Round Steak Varieties ☞ GI = 0.0 (Low)

Veal—Short Loin :Battered + fried ☞ GI = 95 (High)

Veal—Short Loin :braised ☞ GI = 50 (Low)

Veal—Short Loin :Breaded + fried ☞ GI = 95 (High)

Veal—Short Loin :Broiled and/or baked ☞ GI = 0 (Low)

Veal—Short Loin :Fried ☞ GI = 0 (Low)

Veal—Short Loin :Roast ☞ GI = 0 (Low)

Veal—Short Loin :Stewed ☞ GI = 0 (Low)

Veal—Short Loin ☞ GI = 0.0 (Low)

🐄 Veal—Short Ribs :Battered + fried 🐄 GI = 95 (High)

🐄 Veal—Short Ribs :braised 🐄 GI = 50 (Low)

🐄 Veal—Short Ribs :Breaded + fried 🐄 GI = 95 (High)

🐄 Veal—Short Ribs :Broiled and/or baked 🐄 GI = 0 (Low)

🐄 Veal—Short Ribs :Fried 🐄 GI = 0 (Low)

🐄 Veal—Short Ribs :Roast 🐄 GI = 0 (Low)

🐄 Veal—Short Ribs :Stewed 🐄 GI = 0 (Low)

🐄 Veal—Short Ribs 🐄 GI = 0.0 (Low)

🐄 Veal—T-Bone Steak :Battered + fried 🐄 GI = 95 (High)

🐄 Veal—T-Bone Steak :braised 🐄 GI = 50 (Low)

🐄 Veal—T-Bone Steak :Breaded + fried 🐄 GI = 95 (High)

🐄 Veal—T-Bone Steak :Broiled and/or baked 🐄 GI = 0 (Low)

🐄 Veal—T-Bone Steak :Fried 🐄 GI = 0 (Low)

🐄 Veal—T-Bone Steak :Roast 🐄 GI = 0 (Low)

🐄 Veal—T-Bone Steak :Stewed 🐄 GI = 0 (Low)

🐄 Veal—T-Bone Steak 🐄 GI = 0.0 (Low)

🐄 Veal—Tenderloin :Battered + fried 🐄 GI = 95 (High)

🐄 Veal—Tenderloin :braised 🐄 GI = 50 (Low)

🐄 Veal—Tenderloin :Breaded + fried 🐄 GI = 95 (High)

🐄 Veal—Tenderloin :Broiled and/or baked 🐄 GI = 0 (Low)

🐄 Veal—Tenderloin :Fried 🐄 GI = 0 (Low)

🐄 Veal—Tenderloin :Roast 🐄 GI = 0 (Low)

🐄 Veal—Tenderloin :Stewed 🐄 GI = 0 (Low)

Veal—Tenderloin ☛ GI = 0.0 (Low)

Veal—Tongue :Battered + fried ☛ GI = 95 (High)

Veal—Tongue :braised ☛ GI = 50 (Low)

Veal—Tongue :Breaded + fried ☛ GI = 95 (High)

Veal—Tongue :Broiled and/or baked ☛ GI = 0 (Low)

Veal—Tongue :Fried ☛ GI = 0 (Low)

Veal—Tongue ☛ GI = 0.0 (Low)

Veal—Top Sirloin :Battered + fried ☛ GI = 95 (High)

Veal—Top Sirloin :braised ☛ GI = 50 (Low)

Veal—Top Sirloin :Breaded + fried ☛ GI = 95 (High)

Veal—Top Sirloin :Broiled and/or baked ☛ GI = 0 (Low)

Veal—Top Sirloin :Fried ☛ GI = 0 (Low)

Veal—Top Sirloin :Roast ☛ GI = 0 (Low)

Veal—Top Sirloin :Stewed ☛ GI = 0 (Low)

Veal—Top Sirloin ☛ GI = 0.0 (Low)

Veal—Tri-Tip :Battered + fried ☛ GI = 95 (High)

Veal—Tri-Tip :braised ☛ GI = 50 (Low)

Veal—Tri-Tip :Breaded + fried ☛ GI = 95 (High)

Veal—Tri-Tip :Broiled and/or baked ☛ GI = 0 (Low)

Veal—Tri-Tip :Fried ☛ GI = 0 (Low)

Veal—Tri-Tip :Roast ☛ GI = 0 (Low)

Veal—Tri-Tip :Stewed ☛ GI = 0 (Low)

Veal—Tri-Tip ☛ GI = 0.0 (Low)

Veal—Tripe :Battered + fried ☞ GI = 95 (High)

Veal—Tripe :braised ☞ GI = 50 (Low)

Veal—Tripe :Breaded + fried ☞ GI = 95 (High)

Veal—Tripe :Broiled and/or baked ☞ GI = 0 (Low)

Veal—Tripe :Fried ☞ GI = 0 (Low)

Veal—Tripe ☞ GI = 0.0 (Low)

14

BEVERAGES

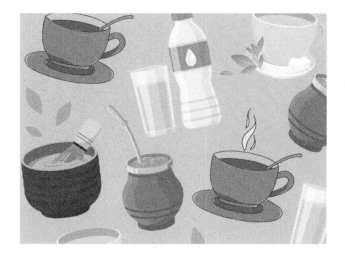

What is the serving size?

The typical serving sizes for low GI beverages are equivalent to:

- 1 cup (8 ounces) 100% vegetable juice
- ¾ cup (6 ounces) 100% fruit juice

- ¾ cup of soft drink
- 1 cup of (8 ounces) milk or yogurt drink

For moderate GI beverages products reduce the serving by 1/3

How Much a Day?

Up to 3 servings per day provided you respect your calorie deficit in your overall daily intake.

Alcoholic Beverage—100 Proof ☛ 0.0 (Low)

Alcoholic Beverage—86 Proof ☛ 0.0 (Low)

Alcoholic Beverage—90 Proof ☛ 0.0 (Low)

Alcoholic Beverage—94 Proof ☛ 0.0 (Low)

Alcoholic Beverage—Amber Hard Cider ☛ 38-44 (Low)

Alcoholic Beverage—Beer ☛ 100 (High)

Alcoholic Beverage—Beer Light Higher Alcohol ☛ 100 (High)

Alcoholic Beverage—Beer Light Low-Carb ☛ 100 (High)

Alcoholic Beverage—Beer Light Regular Alcohol ☛ 100 (High)

Alcoholic Beverage—Beer, lite ☛ 100 (High)

Alcoholic Beverage—Black Russian ☛ 0.0 (Low)

Alcoholic Beverage—Bloody Mary ☛ 31-35 (Low)

Alcoholic Beverage—Brandy ☛ 0.0 (Low)

Alcoholic Beverage—Cabernet Franc ☛ 0 (Low)

Alcoholic Beverage—Cabernet Sauvignon ☛ 0 (Low)

Alcoholic Beverage—Champagne Punch ☞ 0 (Low)

Alcoholic Beverage—Chardonnay ☞ 0 (Low)

Alcoholic Beverage—Chenin Blanc ☞ 0 (Low)

Alcoholic Beverage—Gin ☞ 0.0 (Low)

Alcoholic Beverage—Malt Beverage Sweetened ☞ 88 (High)

Alcoholic Beverage—Pina Colada ☞ 15 (Low)

Alcoholic Beverage—Pina Colada Homemade ☞ 15 (Low)

Alcoholic Beverage—Root Beer, sugar free ☞ 0 (Low)

Alcoholic Beverage—Rum ☞ 0.0 (Low)

Alcoholic Beverage—Sake ☞ 66 (Medium)

Alcoholic Beverage—Sangria ☞ 50 (Low)

Alcoholic Beverage—Tequila ☞ 0.0 (Low)

Alcoholic Beverage—Vodka ☞ 0.0 (Low)

Alcoholic Beverage—Whiskey ☞ 0.0 (Low)

Alcoholic Beverage—Whiskey Sour ☞ 50 (Low)

Alcoholic Beverage—Whiskey Sour Canned ☞ 50 (Low)

Alcoholic Beverage—Wine, red ☞ 0.0 (Low)

Alcoholic Beverage—Wine, white ☞ 0.0 (Low)

Apple cider ☞ 40 (Low)

Cacao powder ☞ 24 (Low)

Carob powder ☞ 41 (Low)

Chicory Beverage ☞ 40 (Low)

Chicory coffee ☞ 0.0 (Low)

Chocolate syrup ☞ 55-68 (Medium)

Chocolate—Ice cream soda ☞ 59.5 (Medium)

Coca Cola ☞ 63 (Medium)

Coca Cola ☞ 63 (Medium)

Cocoa drink— lowfat milk added ☞ 37.5 (Low)

Cocoa drink— milk added ☞ 37 (Low)

Cocoa drink—dry milk, water added ☞ 37.5 (Low)

Cocoa drink—hot chocolate, whole milk ☞ 36 (Low)

Cocoa drink—nonfat milk and low-calorie sweetener ☞ 24 (Low)

Cocoa drink—skim milk added ☞ 37.5 (Low)

Cocoa Drink—whey, lowfat milk added ☞ 24 (Low)

Cocoa drink—whole milk added ☞ 36 (Low)

Cocoa powder ☞ 24 (Low)

Coconut water—fresh ☞ 41 (Low)

Coconut water—packaged ☞ 54 (Low)

Coffee—Bottled or canned ☞ 50 (Low)

Coffee—Brewed ☞ 50 (Low)

Coffee—Brewed Blend Of Decaffeinated ☞ 50 (Low)

Coffee—Brewed Blend Of Regular ☞ 50 (Low)

Coffee—Brewed Espresso Decaffeinated ☞ 50 (Low)

Coffee—Cafe Con Leche ☞ 58 (Medium)

Coffee—Cafe Con Leche Decaffeinated ☞ 58 (Medium)

Coffee—Café Latte (soy milk) ☞ 37 (Low)

Coffee—Cafe Mocha ☛ 58-68 (Medium)

Coffee—Cafe Mocha Decaffeinated ☛ 58-68 (Medium)

Coffee—Cafe Mocha Decaffeinated ☛ 58-68 (Medium)

Coffee—decaffeinated, made from powdered instant ☛ 50 (Low)

Coffee—espresso ☛ 50 (Low)

Coffee—espresso, decaffeinated ☛ 50 (Low)

Coffee—from ground ☛ 50 (Low)

Coffee—from ground decaffeinated ☛ 50 (Low)

Coffee—from ground, 50% regular and 50% decaffeinated ☛ 50 (Low)

Coffee—from ground, regular ☛ 50 (Low)

Coffee—from liquid concentrate ☛ 50 (Low)

Coffee—from powdered instant mix with sugar ☛ 68 (Low)

Coffee—from powdered instant mix, low-calorie sweetener ☛ 27 (Low)

Coffee—from powdered instant mix, with whitener and sugar, instant ☛ 47.5 (Low)

Coffee—instant decaffeinated, and chicory ☛ 50 (Low)

Coffee—latte ☛ 68 (Medium)

Coffee—presweetened with sugar ☛ 66.4 (Medium)

Coffee—rom ground, flavored ☛ 50 (Low)

Cream soda ☛ 55-68 (Medium)

Creamer powder ☛ 16-30 (Low)

Diet beverage ☛ 30-54 (Low)

Diet Coke ☞ 0 (Low)

Diet Cola ☞ 0 (Low)

Diet Green Tea ☞ 0 (Low)

Diet Pepper Cola ☞ 0 (Low)

Drink—Acai Berry Fortified ☞ 24.2 (Low)

Drink—Acai Berry Unsweetned ☞ 24.2 (Low)

Drink—Apricot orange vitamin C added ☞ 47-51 (Low)

Drink—Carbonated citrus ☞ 61-65 (Medium)

Drink—Chocolate-flavored Beverage unsweetened ☞ 50 (Low)

Drink—Cranberry apple juice ☞ 52 (Low)

Drink—Cranberry apple juice low-calorie ☞ 48 (Low)

Drink—Cranberry apple juice vitamin C added ☞ 52 (Low)

Drink—Cranberry juice ☞ 58-61 (Medium)

Drink—Cranberry juice low-calorie ☞ 47-51 (Low)

Drink—Cranberry juice with vitamin C added ☞ 58-61 (Medium)

Drink—Fruit-flavored thirst queencher beverage ☞ 78 (Low)

Drink—Fruit-flavored thirst queencher beverage, low-calorie ☞ 50 (Low)

Drink—Fruit-flavored, from low-calorie powdered mix ☞ 50 (Low)

Drink—Fruit-flavored, from powdered mix ☞ 68 (Medium)

Drink—Fruit-flavored, from sweetened powdered mix ☞ 68 (Medium)

Drink—Fruit-flavored, punches, ades, low-calorie ☞ 50 (Low)

Drink—Grapefruit juice, low-calorie ☞ 50 (Low)

Drink—Grapefruit juice, vitamin C added, low-calorie ☞ 50 (Low)

Drink—Grapefruit Orange juice ☞ 48 (Low)

Drink—Grapefruit Orange juice low-calorie ☞ 47 (Low)

Drink—Milk with chocolate (average) ☞ 37 (Low)

Drink—Milk with chocolate made with skim milk (average) ☞ 37.5 (Low)

Drink—Milk with chocolate made with whole milk (average) ☞ 36 (Low)

Drink—Milk with chocolate, lowfat (average) ☞ 37.5 (Low)

Drink—Orange breakfast ☞ 68 (Medium)

Drink—Orange breakfast from frozen ☞ 68 (Medium)

Drink—Orange breakfast Low-calorie ☞ 50 (Low)

Drink—Orange Cranberry Juice ☞ 49-54 (Low)

Drink—Whey and milk-beverage, Chocolate-flavored ☞ 37.5 (Low)

Espresso—decaffeinated ☞ 0.0 (Low)

Espresso—regular ☞ 0.0 (Low)

Fanta ☞ 68 (Medium)

Ginger beer, sugar-free ☞ 0.0 (Low)

Grape juice, unsweetened ☞ 45 (Low)

Ice cream soda ☞ 64.5 (Medium)

Instant—decaffeinated ☞ 0.0 (Low)

Instant—regular ☞ 0.0 (Low)

Juice— ☛

Juice— ☛

Juice—Aloe Vera ☛ 58-69 (Medium)

Juice—Aloe Vera Vitamin C Fortified ☛ 58-69 (Medium)

Juice—Apple & Raspberry from fresh ☛ 40 (Low)

Juice—Apple cherry ☛ 40-44 (Low)

Juice—Apple cherry ☛ 41-45 (Low)

Juice—Apple grape ☛ 40-44 (Low)

Juice—Apple pear ☛ 40-44 (Low)

Juice—Apple raspberry ☛ 40-44 (Low)

Juice—Apple raspberry grape ☛ 40-44 (Low)

Juice—Apple, 99% —from fresh ☛ 41 (Low)

Juice—Apple, 99% —reconstituted ☛ 50 (Low)

Juice—Apricot ☛ 54 (Low)

Juice—Apricot orange ☛ 47-51 (Low)

Juice—Banana ☛ 58-69 (Medium)

Juice—Carbonated citrus, low-calorie ☛ 49-52 (Low)

Juice—Celery ☛ 32 (Low)

Juice—Cherry ☛ 22-28 (Low)

Juice—Cherry Canned ☛ 22-28 (Low)

Juice—Cranberry apple ☛ 48 (Low)

Juice—Cranberry red grape, unsweetened ☛ 66-69 (Medium)

Juice—Cranberry white grape, unsweetened ☛ 66-69 (Medium)

📖 Juice—Cranberry, unsweetened ☞ 68 (Medium)

📖 Juice—Fruit cocktail ☞ 55 (Low)

📖 Juice—Grape lemon tangerine ☞ 50 (Low)

📖 Juice—Grapefruit and orange ☞ 49 (Low)

📖 Juice—Grapefruit and orange, unsweetened ☞ 49 (Low)

📖 Juice—Grapefruit unsweetened ☞ 48 (Low)

📖 Juice—Orange 25-50% from fresh ☞ 50 (Low)

📖 Juice—Orange and banana ☞ 50 (Low)

📖 Juice—Orange from fresh sweetened with sugar ☞ 60-69 (Medium)

📖 Juice—Orange from fresh unsweetened ☞ 50 (Low)

📖 Juice—Orange from frozen unsweetened ☞ 50 (Low)

📖 Juice—Orange from frozen, with calcium unsweetened ☞ 50 (Low)

📖 Juice—Orange from frozen, with vitamin D unsweetened ☞ 50 (Low)

📖 Juice—Orange juice fresh ☞ 50 (Low)

📖 Juice—Orange peach white grape ☞ 50-54 (Low)

📖 Juice—Orange unsweetened ☞ 50 (Low)

📖 Juice—Orange, 98% reconstituted ☞ 50 (Low)

📖 Juice—Orange, 99% reconstituted ☞ 50 (Low)

📖 Juice—Peach ☞ 38 (Low)

📖 Juice—Peach white grape orange ☞ 50 (Low)

📖 Juice—Pear ☞ 44 (Low)

- Juice—Pineapple apple guava ☛ 43 (Low)

- Juice—Pineapple apple guava with vitamin C ☛ 43 (Low)

- Juice—Pineapple grapefruit, unsweetened ☛ 47 (Low)

- Juice—Pineapple orange banana, unsweetened ☛ 48 (Low)

- Juice—Pineapple orange, unsweetened ☛ 48 (Low)

- Juice—Pineapple unsweetened ☛ 46 (Low)

- Juice—Pineapple with sugar ☛ 60-69 (Medium)

- Juice—Pineapple with vitamin C, unsweetened ☛ 46 (Low)

- Juice—Prune, unsweetened ☛ 45 (Low)

- Juice—Strawberry orange banana, unsweetened ☛ 50 (Low)

- Juice—Tomato ☛ 35 (Low)

- Juice—Tomato and vegetable ☛ 35-38 (Low)

- Lactose-free milk drink ☛ 15-30 (Low)

- Lemonade ☛ 54 (Low)

- Lemonade, low calorie ☛ 16-30 (Low)

- Milk shake with malt ☛ 53 (Low)

- Milk shake—chocolate, made with skim milk ☛ 46.5 (Low)

- Milk shake—flavor or type (average) ☛ 44 (Low)

- Milk shake—flavors other than chocolate, made with skim milk ☛ 46.5 (Low)

- Milk shake—homemade, chocolate ☛ 44 (Low)

- Milk shake—homemade, flavors other than chocolate ☛ 44 (Low)

- Nonalcoholic malt beverage ☛ 40 (Low)

Orange juice, No added Sugar (reconstituted) ☞ 50 (Low)

Protein supplement, plant-based ☞ 28-44 (Low)

Rice beverage ☞ 100 (High)

Soft drink— sugar-free ☞ 50 (Low)

Soft drink—average ☞ 63-69 (Medium)

Soft drink—cola-type ☞ 63-69 (Medium)

Soft drink—cola-type, decaffeinated ☞ 63-69 (Medium)

Soft drink—cola-type, high amount of caffeine ☞ 63-69 (Medium)

Soft drink—cola-type, sugar free, decaffeinated ☞ 50 (Low)

Soft drink—cola-type, sugar-free ☞ 50 (Low)

Soft drink—fruit flavored with caffeine ☞ 63-69 (Medium)

Soft drink—fruit flavored, sugar free, with caffeine ☞ 50 (Low)

Soft drink—fruit-flavored ☞ 63-69 (Medium)

Soft drink—pepper-type, sugar free ☞ 50 (Low)

Soft drink—pepper-type, sugar free and decaffeinated, ☞ 50 (Low)

Soft drink—sugar free, fruit-flavored ☞ 50 (Low)

Soft drink, cola-type ☞ 58-69 (Medium)

Tea black—leaf, unsweetened ☞ Low

Tea herbal—from chicory roots, ginger ☞ Low

Tea herbal—from dried mint, lemon and ginger ☞ Low

Tea herbal—from fresh mint, lemon and ginger ☞ Low

Tea with fennel—made up with water ☞ Low

Tea with licorice—made up with water ☞ Low

Tea—Black Brewed 🖝 0 (Low)

Tea—Black Ready to drink 🖝 0 (Low)

Tea—chamomile 🖝 Low

Tea—green, leaf, unsweetened 🖝 Low

Water—Bottled 🖝 0 (Low)

15

BREADS & BAKERY PRODUCTS

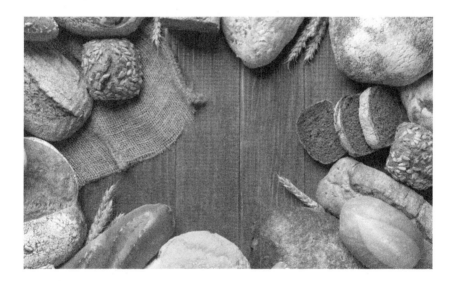

What is the serving size?

The typical serving size for low GI breads and bakery products is equivalent to:

- 1 slice bread

- ½ of muffin, bagel, or hamburger bun
- ½ slice of bakery products
- ½ cup cereal

For moderate GI breads and bakery products reduce the serving by 1/3

How Much a Day?

Up to 8 servings per day

Bagel ☛ 72 (High)

Bagel chip ☛ 72 (High)

Bagel—multigrain ☛ 43 (Low)

Bagel—multigrain, toasted ☛ 43 (Low)

Bagel—multigrain, with raisins ☛ 43 (Low)

Bagel—multigrain, with raisins, toasted ☛ 43 (Low)

Bagel—oat bran ☛ 47 (Low)

Bagel—oat bran, toasted ☛ 47 (Low)

Bagel—pumpernickel ☛ 50 (Low)

Bagel—pumpernickel, toasted ☛ 50 (Low)

Bagel—toasted ☛ 72 (High)

Bagel—wheat ☛ 71 (High)

Bagel—wheat, toasted ☛ 71 (High)

Bagel—wheat, with fruit and nuts ☛ 71 (High)

Bagel—wheat, with fruit and nuts, toasted ☛ 71 (High)

Bagel—wheat, with raisins ☛ 71 (High)

Bagel—wheat, with raisins, toasted ☛ 71 (High)

Bagel—whole wheat, 100% ☛ 71 (High)

Bagel—whole wheat, 100%, toasted ☛ 71 (High)

Bagel—whole wheat, 100%, with raisins ☛ 71 (High)

Bagel—whole wheat, 100%, with raisins, toasted ☛ 71 (High)

Bagel—whole wheat, other than 100% or NS as to 100% ☛ 71 (High)

Bagel—whole wheat, other than 100% or NS as to 100%, toasted ☛ 71 (High)

Bagel—with fruit other than raisins ☛ 72 (High)

Bagel—with fruit other than raisins, toasted ☛ 72 (High)

Bagel—with raisins ☛ 72 (High)

Bagel—with raisins, toasted ☛ 72 (High)

Baklava ☛ 59 (Medium)

Bread—100% Whole Grain ☛ 51 (Low)

Bread stick—hard, low sodium ☛ 70 (High)

Bread stick—hard, whole wheat ☛ 83 (High)

Bread stick—average hard or soft ☛ 70 (High)

Bread stick—soft ☛ 70 (High)

Bread stick—soft, made with parmesan cheese, garlic ☛ 70 (High)

Bread sticks—hard ☛ 70 (High)

Bread stuffing ☛ 74 (High)

Bread stuffing—made with egg ☛ 74 (High)

Bread—barley ☞ 67 (Medium)

Bread—black ☞ 76 (High)

Bread—black, toasted ☞ 76 (High)

Bread—cinnamon ☞ 70 (High)

Bread—cinnamon, toasted ☞ 73 (High)

Bread—Cuban ☞ 95 (High)

Bread—Cuban, toasted ☞ 95 (High)

Bread—dough, fried ☞ 66 (High)

Bread—French or Vienna ☞ 95 (High)

Bread—French or Vienna, toasted ☞ 95 (High)

Bread—French or Vienna, whole wheat, avergae home recipe ☞ 71 (High)

Bread—French or Vienna, whole wheat, average purchased at bakery, toasted ☞ 71 (High)

Bread—fruit and nut ☞ 57.9 (Medium)

Bread—fruit, without nuts ☞ 57.9 (Medium)

Bread—garlic ☞ 95 (High)

Bread—garlic, toasted ☞ 95 (High)

Bread—Italian, Grecian, Armenian ☞ 70 (High)

Bread—Italian, Grecian, Armenian, toasted ☞ 73 (High)

Bread—lowfat, 98% fat free ☞ 95 (High)

Bread—lowfat, 98% fat free, toasted ☞ 95 (High)

Bread—made from home recipe or purchased at a bakery, NS as to major flour ☞ 70 (High)

Bread—made from home recipe or purchased at a bakery, toasted, NS as to major flour ☞ 73 (High)

Bread—marble rye and pumpernickel ☞ 50 (Low)

Bread—marble rye and pumpernickel, toasted ☞ 50 (Low)

Bread—multigrain ☞ 43 (Low)

Bread—multigrain, reduced calorie and/or high fiber ☞ 43 (Low)

Bread—multigrain, reduced calorie and/or high fiber, toasted ☞ 43 (Low)

Bread—multigrain, toasted ☞ 43 (Low)

Bread—multigrain, with raisins ☞ 43 (Low)

Bread—multigrain, with raisins, toasted ☞ 43 (Low)

Bread—Native, Puerto Rican style ☞ 70 (High)

Bread—Native, Puerto Rican style, toasted ☞ 73 (High)

Bread—NS as to major flour ☞ 70 (High)

Bread—nut ☞ 57.9 (Medium)

Bread—oat bran ☞ 31 (Low)

Bread—oat bran, reduced calorie and/or high fiber ☞ 31 (Low)

Bread—oat bran, reduced calorie and/or high fiber, toasted ☞ 31 (Low)

Bread—oat bran, toasted ☞ 31 (Low)

Bread—oatmeal ☞ 55 (Low)

Bread—oatmeal, toasted ☞ 55 (Low)

Bread—pita ☞ 57 (Medium)

Bread—pita, toasted ☞ 57 (Medium)

Bread—pita, wheat or cracked wheat ☞ 53 (Low)

Bread—pita, wheat or cracked wheat, toasted ☞ 53 (Low)

Bread—pita, whole wheat, 100% ☞ 71 (High)

Bread—pita, whole wheat, 100%, toasted ☞ 71 (High)

Bread—pita, whole wheat, average ☞ 71 (High)

Bread—pita, whole wheat, average ☞ 71 (High)

Bread—pumpernickel ☞ 50 (Low)

Bread—pumpernickel, toasted ☞ 50 (Low)

Bread—pumpkin ☞ 57.9 (Medium)

Bread—raisin ☞ 63 (Medium)

Bread—raisin, toasted ☞ 63 (Medium)

Bread—reduced calorie and/or high fiber, Italian ☞ 68 (Medium)

Bread—reduced calorie and/or high fiber, Italian, toasted ☞ 68 (Medium)

Bread—reduced calorie and/or high fiber, white or NFS ☞ 68 (Medium)

Bread—reduced calorie, white or NFS, toasted and/or high fiber, ☞ 68 (Medium)

Bread—white or NFS, reduced calorie with fruit and/or nuts, and/or high fiber ☞ 68 (Medium)

Bread—reduced calorie and/or high fiber, white or NFS, with fruit and/or nuts, toasted ☞ 68 (Medium)

Bread—rice, toasted ☞ 66.5 (Medium)

Bread—rye ☞ 58 (Medium)

Bread—rye, reduced calorie and/or high fiber ☞ 68 (Medium)

Bread—rye, reduced calorie and/or high fiber, toasted ☞ 68 (Medium)

Bread—rye, toasted ☞ 58 (Medium)

Bread—sour dough ☞ 54 (Low)

Bread—sour dough, toasted ☞ 54 (Low)

Bread—sprouted wheat, toasted ☞ 53 (Low)

Bread—sunflower meal ☞ 57 (Medium)

Bread—wheat bran ☞ 71 (High)

Bread—wheat bran, toasted ☞ 71 (High)

Bread—wheat or cracked wheat ☞ 71 (High)

Bread—wheat or cracked wheat, made from home recipe or purchased at bakery ☞ 53 (Low)

Bread—wheat or cracked wheat, made from home recipe or purchased at bakery, toasted ☞ 53 (Low)

Bread—wheat or cracked wheat, reduced calorie and/or high fiber ☞ 71 (High)

Bread—wheat or cracked wheat, reduced calorie and/or high fiber, toasted ☞ 71 (High)

Bread—wheat or cracked wheat, toasted ☞ 71 (High)

Bread—wheat or cracked wheat, with raisins ☞ 53 (Low)

Bread—wheat or cracked wheat, with raisins, toasted ☞ 53 (Low)

Bread—white ☞ 70 (High)

Bread—white with whole wheat swirl ☞ 70 (High)

Bread—white with whole wheat swirl, toasted ☞ 70 (High)

Bread—white, low sodium or no salt ☞ 70 (High)

Bread—white, low sodium or no salt, toasted ☛ 73 (High)

Bread—white, made from home recipe or purchased at a bakery ☛ 70 (High)

Bread—white, made from home recipe or purchased at a bakery, toasted ☛ 73 (High)

Bread—white, special formula, added fiber ☛ 68 (Medium)

Bread—white, toasted ☛ 73 (High)

Bread—whole wheat, 100% ☛ 71 (High)

Bread—whole wheat, 100%, made from home recipe or purchased at bakery ☛ 71 (High)

Bread—whole wheat, 100%, made from home recipe or purchased at bakery, toasted ☛ 71 (High)

Bread—whole wheat, 100%, toasted ☛ 71 (High)

Bread—whole wheat, 100%, with raisins ☛ 71 (High)

Bread—whole wheat, 100%, with raisins, toasted ☛ 71 (High)

Bread—whole wheat, NS as to 100%, with raisins ☛ 71 (High)

Bread—whole wheat, NS as to 100%, with raisins, toasted ☛ 71 (High)

Bread—whole wheat, other than 100% or NS as to 100% ☛ 71 (High)

Bread—whole wheat, other than 100% or NS as to 100%, made from home recipe or purchased at bakery ☛ 71 (High)

Bread—whole wheat, other than 100% or NS as to 100%, made from home recipe or purchased at bakery, toasted ☛ 71 (High)

Bread—whole wheat, other than 100% or NS as to 100%, toasted ☛ 71 (High)

🌾 Bread—zucchini 🖝 57.9 (Medium)

🌾 Cake—prepared with glutinous rice 🖝 64 (Medium)

🌾 Cake—angel food, NS as to icing 🖝 67 (Medium)

🌾 Cake—angel food, with fruit and icing or filling 🖝 67 (Medium)

🌾 Cake—angel food, with icing 🖝 67 (Medium)

🌾 Cake—angel food, without icing 🖝 67 (Medium)

🌾 Cake—applesauce, NS as to icing 🖝 44 (Low)

🌾 Cake—applesauce, with icing 🖝 44 (Low)

🌾 Cake—applesauce, without icing 🖝 44 (Low)

🌾 Cake—banana, NS as to icing 🖝 47 (Low)

🌾 Cake—banana, with icing 🖝 47 (Low)

🌾 Cake—banana, without icing 🖝 47 (Low)

🌾 Cake—black forest made with chocolate and cherry 🖝 38 (Low)

🌾 Cake—butter, with icing 🖝 42 (Low)

🌾 Cake—butter, without icing 🖝 42 (Low)

🌾 Cake—carrot, average for icing 🖝 62 (Medium)

🌾 Cake—carrot, with icing 🖝 62 (Medium)

🌾 Cake—carrot, without icing 🖝 62 (Medium)

🌾 Cake—chocolate, made from home recipe, average for icing 🖝 38 (Low)

🌾 Cake—chocolate, pudding type mix with light icing, light coating or light filling 🖝 38 (Low)

🌾 Cake—chocolate, pudding-type mix (oil, eggs, and water added to dry mix), icing not specified 🖝 38 (Low)

Cake—chocolate, pudding-type mix, with icing, filling or coating 38 (Low)

Cake—chocolate, pudding-type mix, without icing or filling 38 (Low)

Cake—chocolate, pudding-type mix, made by "Lite" recipe with filling, icing, or coating 38 (Low)

Cake—chocolate, standard-type mix, with filling, icing, or coating 38 (Low)

Cake—chocolate, standard-type mix, without icing or filling 38 (Low)

Cake—chocolate, with icing, coating, or filling, prepared from home recipe 38 (Low)

Cake—chocolate, with icing, coating, or filling, purchased ready-to-eat 38 (Low)

Cake—chocolate, without icing or filling, prepared from home recipe 38 (Low)

Cake—chocolate, without icing or filling, purchased ready-to-eat 38 (Low)

Cake—chocolate, with icing, light 38 (Low)

Cake—coconut, with icing 42 (Low)

Cake—cupCake, chocolate, icing not specified 38 (Low)

Cake—cupCake, chocolate, with icing or filling 38 (Low)

Cake—cupCake, chocolate, fruit filling or cream filling 38 (Low)

Cake—cupCake, chocolate, without icing or filling 38 (Low)

Cake—cupCake, not chocolate, icing not specified (average) 57.5 (Medium)

Cake—cupCake, not chocolate, with cream and fruit filling ☞ 57.5 (Medium)

Cake—cupCake, not chocolate, with icing or filling ☞ 57.5 (Medium)

Cake—cupCake—not chocolate, with icing or filling, lowfat, cholesterol free ☞ 73 (High)

Cake—cupCake—not chocolate, without icing or filling ☞ 57.5 (Medium)

Cake—cupCake—NS as to type or icing ☞ 42 (Low)

Cake—cupCake—NS as to type, with icing ☞ 42 (Low)

Cake—Dobos Torte (non-chocolate layer cake with chocolate filling and icing) ☞ 38 (Low)

Cake—frozen yogurt and cake layer, chocolate, with icing ☞ 49.5 (Low)

Cake—fruit Cake—light or dark, holiday type cake ☞ 57.9 (Medium)

Cake—German chocolate, with icing and filling ☞ 38 (Low)

Cake—gingerbread, without icing ☞ 57.9 (Medium)

Cake—ice cream and cake roll, chocolate ☞ 49.5 (Low)

Cake—ice cream and cake roll, not chocolate ☞ 51.5 (Low)

Cake—lemon, lowfat, with icing ☞ 42 (Low)

Cake—lemon, lowfat, without icing ☞ 42 (Low)

Cake—lemon, NS as to icing ☞ 42 (Low)

Cake—lemon, with icing ☞ 42 (Low)

Cake—lemon, without icing ☞ 42 (Low)

Cake—marble, with icing ☞ 40 (Low)

🍰 Cake—marble, without icing ☛ 40 (Low)

🍰 Cake—NS as to type, with or without icing ☛ 42 (Low)

🍰 Cake—nut, NS as to icing ☛ 42 (Low)

🍰 Cake—nut, with icing ☛ 42 (Low)

🍰 Cake—nut, without icing ☛ 42 (Low)

🍰 Cake—plum pudding ☛ 57.9 (Medium)

🍰 Cake—poppyseed, without icing ☛ 42 (Low)

🍰 Cake—pound, chocolate ☛ 54 (Low)

🍰 Cake—pound, chocolate, fat free, cholesterol free ☛ 54 (Low)

🍰 Cake—pound, fat free, cholesterol free ☛ 54 (Low)

🍰 Cake—pound, reduced fat, cholesterol free ☛ 54 (Low)

🍰 Cake—pound, with icing ☛ 54 (Low)

🍰 Cake—pound, without icing ☛ 54 (Low)

🍰 Cake—pumpkin, NS as to icing ☛ 62 (Medium)

🍰 Cake—pumpkin, with icing ☛ 62 (Medium)

🍰 Cake—pumpkin, without icing ☛ 62 (Medium)

🍰 Cake—raisin-nut, without icing ☛ 54 (Low)

🍰 Cake—spice, NS as to icing ☛ 42 (Low)

🍰 Cake—spice, with icing ☛ 42 (Low)

🍰 Cake—spice, without icing ☛ 42 (Low)

🍰 Cake—sponge, chocolate, with icing ☛ 87 (High)

🍰 Cake—sponge, with icing ☛ 46 (Low)

🍰 Cake—sponge, without icing ☛ 46 (Low)

Cake—upside down (all fruits) ☞ 44 (Low)

Cake—white, made from home recipe or purchased ready-to-eat, NS as to icing ☞ 42 (Low)

Cake—white, pudding-type mix (oil, egg whites, and water added to dry mix), NS as to icing ☞ 42 (Low)

Cake—white, pudding-type mix (oil, egg whites, and water added to dry mix), with icing ☞ 42 (Low)

Cake—white, pudding-type mix (oil, egg whites, and water added to dry mix), without icing ☞ 42 (Low)

Cake—white, standard-type mix (egg whites and water added to mix), with icing ☞ 42 (Low)

Cake—white, standard-type mix (egg whites and water added to mix), without icing ☞ 42 (Low)

Cake—white, standard-type mix (egg whites and water added), NS as to icing ☞ 42 (Low)

Cake—white, with icing, made from home recipe or purchased ready-to-eat ☞ 42 (Low)

Cake—white, without icing, made from home recipe or purchased ready-to-eat ☞ 42 (Low)

Cake—yellow, made from home recipe or purchased ready-to- eat, NS as to icing ☞ 42 (Low)

Cake—yellow, pudding-type mix (oil, eggs, and water added to dry mix), NS as to icing ☞ 42 (Low)

Cake—yellow, pudding-type mix (oil, eggs, and water added to dry mix), with icing ☞ 42 (Low)

Cake—yellow, pudding-type mix (oil, eggs, and water added to dry mix), without icing ☞ 42 (Low)

Cake—yellow, standard-type mix (eggs and water added to dry

mix), NS as to icing ☞ 42 (Low)

🌿 Cake—yellow, standard-type mix (eggs and water added to dry mix), with icing ☞ 42 (Low)

🌿 Cake—yellow, standard-type mix (eggs and water added to dry mix), without icing ☞ 42 (Low)

🌿 Cake—yellow, with icing, made from home recipe or purchased ready-to-eat ☞ 42 (Low)

🌿 Cake—yellow, without icing, made from home recipe or purchased ready-to-eat ☞ 42 (Low)

🌿 Cake—zucchini, with icing ☞ 57.9 (Medium)

🌿 Cake—zucchini, without icing ☞ 57.9 (Medium)

🌿 Cheesecake—Common ☞ 50 (Low)

🌿 Cheesecake—with fruit ☞ 50 (Low)

🌿 Cheesecake—chocolate ☞ 50 (Low)

🌿 Cheesecake—chocolate, low fat ☞ 50 (Low)

🌿 Cheesecake—diet ☞ 50 (Low)

🌿 Cheesecake—diet, made with fruit ☞ 50 (Low)

🌿 Churros ☞ 76 (High)

🌿 Cobbler—apple from frozen ☞ 46 (Low)

🌿 Cobbler—apple from fresh ☞ 46 (Low)

🌿 Cobbler—berry ☞ 59 (Medium)

🌿 Cobbler—cherry ☞ 55 (Low)

🌿 Cobbler—peach ☞ 55 (Low)

🌿 Cobbler—pineapple ☞ 59 (Medium)

🌿 Cobbler—Apple Pomegranate ☞ 51 (Low)

🍃 Cobbler—Plum ☛ 58 (Medium)

🍃 Cobbler—Blueberry ☛ 56 (Medium)

🍃 Cobbler—Peach-Lavender ☛ 58 (Medium)

🍃 Cobbler—Strawberry Buttermilk ☛ 57 (Medium)

🍃 Cobbler—Mixed-Fruit ☛ 59 (Medium)

🍃 Cobbler—Peach Apricot ☛ 57 (Medium)

🍃 Coffee cake—crumb ☛ 58 (Medium)

🍃 Coffee cake—crumb cheese-filled ☛ 58 (Medium)

🍃 Coffee cake—quick-bread type or crumb, custard filled ☛ 58 (Medium)

🍃 Coffee cake—crumb, low fat, cholesterol-free ☛ 58 (Medium)

🍃 Coffee cake—crumb, with fruit ☛ 58 (Medium)

🍃 Coffee cake—crumb, with icing ☛ 58 (Medium)

🍃 Coffee cake—Common ☛ 58 (Medium)

🍃 Coffee cake—yeast type ☛ 58 (Medium)

🍃 Coffee cake—yeast type, fat-free, prepared with fruit ☛ 58 (Medium)

🍃 Coffee cake—yeast type, purchased at a bakery ☛ 58 (Medium)

🍃 Coffee cake—yeast type, prepared from home recipe ☛ 58 (Medium)

🍃 Corn flour—patty, fried ☛ 75.5 (High)

🍃 Corn flour—tart, fried ☛ 75.5 (High)

🍃 Corn pone—baked ☛ 75.5 (High)

🍃 Cornbread—muffin, round, stick ☛ 75.5 (High)

Cornbread—muffin, made from home recipe 🖙 75.5 (High)

Cornbread—muffin, purchased at a bakery 🖙 75.5 (High)

Cornbread—muffin, round, stick, toasted 🖙 75.5 (High)

Cornbread—stuffing 🖙 75.5 (High)

Cornbread—prepared from home recipe 🖙 75.5 (High)

Cornbread—made from mix 🖙 75.5 (High)

Cream puff, eclair, custard or cream filled, iced 🖙 59 (Medium)

Cream puff, eclair, custard or cream filled, iced, reduced fat 🖙 59 (Medium)

Cream puff, eclair, custard or cream filled, not iced 🖙 59 (Medium)

Cream puff, eclair, custard or cream filled, NS as to icing 🖙 59 (Medium)

Crepe, plain 🖙 67 (Medium)

Crisp, apple, apple dessert 🖙 48.7 (Low)

Crisp, cherry 🖙 59 (Medium)

Crisp, peach 🖙 59 (Medium)

Crisp, rhubarb 🖙 59 (Medium)

Crispbread, rye, no added fat 🖙 64 (Medium)

Crispbread, wheat or rye, extra crispy 🖙 64 (Medium)

Crispbread, wheat, no added fat 🖙 55 (Medium)

Croissant 🖙 67 (Medium)

Croissant, cheese 🖙 67 (Medium)

Croissant, chocolate 🖙 67 (Medium)

🍃 Croissant, fruit ☛ 67 (Medium)

🍃 Cruller ☛ 76 (High)

🍃 Crumpet ☛ 69 (Medium)

🍃 Crumpet, toasted ☛ 69 (Medium)

🍃 Danish pastry, plain or spice ☛ 59 (Medium)

🍃 Danish pastry, with cheese ☛ 59 (Medium)

🍃 Danish pastry, with cheese, fat free, cholesterol free ☛ 59 (Medium)

🍃 Danish pastry, with fruit ☛ 59 (Medium)

🍃 Danish pastry, with nuts ☛ 59 (Medium)

🍃 Doughnut—cake type ☛ 76 (High)

🍃 Doughnut—cake type, chocolate ☛ 76 (High)

🍃 Doughnut—cake style, chocolate covered ☛ 76 (High)

🍃 Doughnut—cake style, chocolate covered, with peanuts ☛ 76 (High)

🍃 Doughnut—cake style, chocolate, with chocolate icing ☛ 76 (High)

🍃 Doughnut—chocolate cream-filled ☛ 76 (High)

🍃 Doughnut—custard-filled ☛ 76 (High)

🍃 Doughnut—custard-filled, with icing ☛ 76 (High)

🍃 Doughnut—jelly ☛ 76 (High)

🍃 Doughnut—Not specified type cake or yeast (average) ☛ 76 (High)

🍃 Doughnut—oriental ☛ 76 (High)

🍃 Doughnut—raised or yeast ☛ 76 (High)

Doughnut—raised or yeast, chocolate ☛ 76 (High)

Doughnut—raised or yeast, chocolate covered ☛ 76 (High)

Doughnut—raised or yeast, chocolate, with chocolate icing ☛ 76 (High)

Doughnut—wheat ☛ 76 (High)

Empanada—Mexican style, pumpkin ☛ 59 (Medium)

French cruller ☛ 76 (High)

French toast sticks, plain ☛ 67 (Medium)

French toast, plain ☛ 67 (Medium)

Fritter, apple ☛ 59 (Medium)

Hush puppy ☛ 75.5 (High)

Bread—Ethiopian style, injera ☛ 72 (High)

Bread—Swedish flatbread ☛ 79 (High)

Bread—Turkish bread ☛ 87 (High)

Bread—Lebanese flatbread ☛ 97 (High)

Muffin—bran with fruit, lowfat ☛ 60 (Medium)

Muffin—bran with fruit, no fat, no cholesterol ☛ 60 (Medium)

Muffin—carrot ☛ 62 (Medium)

Muffin—chocolate ☛ 53 (Low)

Muffin—chocolate chip ☛ 53 (Low)

Muffin—English ☛ 77 (High)

Muffin—English, multigrain ☛ 43 (Low)

Muffin—English, multigrain, toasted ☛ 43 (Low)

Muffin—English, oat bran, toasted ☛ 47 (Low)

Muffin—English, toasted ☛ 77 (High)

Muffin—English, wheat bran ☛ 71 (High)

Muffin—English, wheat bran, toasted ☛ 71 (High)

Muffin—English, wheat or cracked wheat ☛ 71 (High)

Muffin—English, wheat or cracked wheat, toasted ☛ 71 (High)

Muffin—English, wheat or cracked wheat, with raisins, toasted ☛ 71 (High)

Muffin—English, whole-wheat, 100%, toasted ☛ 71 (High)

Muffin—English, whole-wheat, 100%, with raisins, toasted ☛ 71 (High)

Muffin—English, whole-wheat (average) ☛ 71 (High)

Muffin—English, whole-wheat, with raisins, toasted ☛ 71 (High)

Muffin—English, with fruit other than raisins, toasted ☛ 77 (High)

Muffin—English, with raisins ☛ 77 (High)

Muffin—English, with raisins, toasted ☛ 77 (High)

Muffin—fruit and/or nuts ☛ 59 (Medium)

Muffin—fruit, fat free, cholesterol free ☛ 59 (Medium)

Muffin—multigrain, with nuts ☛ 64.5 (Medium)

Muffin—Common ☛ 61.1 (Medium)

Muffin—oat bran ☛ 60 (Medium)

Muffin—oat bran with fruit and/or nuts ☛ 60 (Medium)

Muffin—oatmeal ☛ 69 (Medium)

Muffin—plain ☛ 44 (Low)

Muffin—pumpkin ☛ 62 (Medium)

Muffin—wheat ☛ 60 (Medium)

Muffin—wheat bran ☛ 60 (Medium)

Muffin—whole wheat ☛ 60 (Medium)

Muffin—zucchini ☛ 57.9 (Medium)

Pancakes—buckwheat ☛ 102 (High)

Pancakes—cornmeal ☛ 67 (Medium)

Pancakes—plain ☛ 67 (Medium)

Pancakes—reduced calorie, high fiber ☛ 67 (Medium)

Pancakes—sour dough ☛ 67 (Medium)

Pancakes—whole-wheat ☛ 67 (Medium)

Pancakes—with fruit ☛ 67 (Medium)

Pastry—fruit-filled ☛ 59 (Medium)

Pastry—Italian, with cheese ☛ 59 (Medium)

Pastry—mainly flour, almond and water, fried ☛ 59 (Medium)

Pastry—mainly flour and water, fried ☛ 59 (Medium)

Pastry—Oriental, prepared with almond paste filling, fried ☛ 59 (Medium)

Pastry—Oriental, prepared with almond paste filling, baked ☛ 59 (Medium)

Pastry—Oriental, prepared with bean paste, fried ☛ 59 (Medium)

Pastry—Oriental, prepared with bean paste, baked ☛ 59 (Medium)

Pastry—puff ☛ 59 (Medium)

Pastry—puff, custard or cream filled, icing not specified ☛ 59 (Medium)

Pie—apple, diet ☛ 59 (Medium)

Pie—apple, fried ☛ 59 (Medium)

Pie—apple ☛ 59 (Medium)

Pie—apple, one crust ☛ 59 (Medium)

Pie—apple, two crusts ☛ 59 (Medium)

Pie—apricot, fried ☛ 59 (Medium)

Pie—apricot, two crusts ☛ 59 (Medium)

Pie—banana cream ☛ 59 (Medium)

Pie—berry ☛ 59 (Medium)

Pie—blackberry, two crusts ☛ 59 (Medium)

Pie—blueberry ☛ 59 (Medium)

Pie—blueberry, one crust ☛ 59 (Medium)

Pie—blueberry, two crusts ☛ 59 (Medium)

Pie—buttermilk ☛ 59 (Medium)

Pie—cherry, fried ☛ 59 (Medium)

Pie—cherry ☛ 59 (Medium)

Pie—cherry, prepared with sour cream and/or cream cheese ☛ 59 (Medium)

Pie—cherry, one crust ☛ 59 (Medium)

Pie—cherry, two crusts ☛ 59 (Medium)

Pie—chess ☛ 59 (Medium)

Pie—chocolate cream ☛ 59 (Medium)

Pie—chocolate cream ☛ 59 (Medium)

Pie—chocolate marshmallow ☛ 59 (Medium)

Pie—coconut cream ☞ 59 (Medium)

Pie—coconut cream ☞ 59 (Medium)

Pie—custard ☞ 59 (Medium)

Pie—individual size or tart ☞ 59 (Medium)

Pie—lemon (not cream) ☞ 59 (Medium)

Pie—lemon (not merinue) ☞ 59 (Medium)

Pie—lemon cream ☞ 59 (Medium)

Pie—lemon meringue ☞ 59 (Medium)

Pie—mince ☞ 59 (Medium)

Pie—mince, two crusts ☞ 59 (Medium)

Pie—Common ☞ 59 (Medium)

Pie—oatmeal ☞ 59 (Medium)

Pie—peach, fried ☞ 59 (Medium)

Pie—peach ☞ 59 (Medium)

Pie—peach, one crust ☞ 59 (Medium)

Pie—peach, two crusts ☞ 59 (Medium)

Pie—peanut butter cream ☞ 59 (Medium)

Pie—pecan ☞ 59 (Medium)

Pie—pineapple cream ☞ 59 (Medium)

Pie—pineapple ☞ 59 (Medium)

Pie—pineapple, two crusts ☞ 59 (Medium)

Pie—plum, two crusts ☞ 59 (Medium)

Pie—praline mousse ☞ 59 (Medium)

Pie—prune, one crust ☞ 59 (Medium)

Pie—pudding ☞ 59 (Medium)

Pie—pudding, with chocolate coating ☞ 59 (Medium)

Pie—pumpkin ☞ 59 (Medium)

Pie—raisin ☞ 59 (Medium)

Pie—raisin, two crusts ☞ 59 (Medium)

Pie—raspberry, one crust ☞ 59 (Medium)

Pie—raspberry, two crusts ☞ 59 (Medium)

Pie—rhubarb, one crust ☞ 59 (Medium)

Pie—rhubarb, two crusts ☞ 59 (Medium)

Pie—squash ☞ 59 (Medium)

Pie—strawberry cream ☞ 59 (Medium)

Pie—strawberry, one crust ☞ 59 (Medium)

Pie—strawberry rhubarb, two crusts ☞ 59 (Medium)

Pie—sweetpotato ☞ 59 (Medium)

Pie—vanilla cream ☞ 59 (Medium)

Roll—French or Vienna ☞ 95 (High)

Roll—French or Vienna, toasted ☞ 95 (High)

Roll—garlic ☞ 73 (High)

Roll—hard, NS as to major flour ☞ 73 (High)

Roll—hoagie, submarine ☞ 73 (High)

Roll—hoagie, submarine, toasted ☞ 73 (High)

Roll—made from home recipe or purchased at a bakery, NS as to major flour ☞ 70 (High)

Roll—Mexican, bolillo ☛ 73 (High)

Roll—multigrain ☛ 43 (Low)

Roll—multigrain, toasted ☛ 43 (Low)

Roll—NS as to major flour ☛ 70 (High)

Roll—NS as to major flour, toasted ☛ 73 (High)

Roll—pumpernickel ☛ 50 (Low)

Roll—pumpernickel, toasted ☛ 50 (Low)

Roll—rye ☛ 58 (Medium)

Roll—sour dough ☛ 54 (Low)

Roll—sweet ☛ 57.9 (Medium)

Roll—sweet, cinnamon bun, frosted ☛ 57.9 (Medium)

Roll—sweet, cinnamon bun, no frosting ☛ 57.9 (Medium)

Roll—sweet, crumb topping, Mexican (Pan Dulce) ☛ 59 (Medium)

Roll—sweet, no topping, Mexican (Pan Dulce) ☛ 59 (Medium)

Roll—sweet, sugar topping, Mexican (Pan Dulce) ☛ 59 (Medium)

Roll—sweet, toasted ☛ 57.9 (Medium)

Roll—sweet, with fruit and nuts, frosted ☛ 57.9 (Medium)

Roll—sweet, with fruit, frosted ☛ 57.9 (Medium)

Roll—sweet, with fruit, frosted, diet ☛ 57.9 (Medium)

Roll—sweet, with fruit, frosted, fat free ☛ 57.9 (Medium)

Roll—sweet, with fruit, no frosting ☛ 57.9 (Medium)

Roll—sweet, with nuts, frosted ☛ 57.9 (Medium)

Roll—sweet, with nuts, no frosting ☛ 57.9 (Medium)

Roll—wheat or cracked wheat 🖝 71 (High)

Roll—wheat or cracked wheat, made from home recipe or purchased at bakery 🖝 71 (High)

Roll—white, hard 🖝 73 (High)

Roll—white, hard, toasted 🖝 73 (High)

Roll—white, soft 🖝 70 (High)

Roll—white, soft, prepared from home recipe 🖝 70 (High)

Roll—white, soft, purchased at a bakery 🖝 70 (High)

Roll—white, soft, and/or high fiber 🖝 68 (Medium)

Roll—white, soft, and/or high fiber, toasted 🖝 68 (Medium)

Roll—white, soft, toasted 🖝 70 (High)

Roll—whole wheat, 100% 🖝 71 (High)

Roll—whole-wheat, 100%, prepared from home recipe 🖝 71 (High)

Roll—whole-wheat, 100%, purchased at bakery 🖝 71 (High)

Roll—whole-wheat, 100%, toasted 🖝 71 (High)

Roll—whole-wheat, not specified as to 100% (average) 🖝 71 (High)

Roll—whole-wheat, not specified as to 100%, toasted 🖝 71 (High)

Roll—whole-wheat, other than 100%, prepared from home recipe 🖝 71 (High)

Roll—whole-wheat, other than 100%, purchased at bakery 🖝 71 (High)

Roll—whole wheat, prepared from home recipe 🖝 71 (High)

Roll—whole wheat, purchased at bakery 🖝 71 (High)

Roll—whole wheat, prepared from home recipe, toasted ☞ 71 (High)

Roll—whole wheat, purchased at bakery, toasted ☞ 71 (High)

Roll—wheat or cracked wheat, toasted ☞ 71 (High)

Roll—wheat or cracked wheat ☞ 71 (High)

Sopaipilla—without syrup or honey ☞ 59 (Medium)

Strudel—apple ☞ 59 (Medium)

Strudel—berry ☞ 59 (Medium)

Strudel—cherry ☞ 59 (Medium)

Strudel—fruits ☞ 59 (Medium)

Tamale—sweet, with fruit ☞ 59 (Medium)

Turnover or dumpling—apple ☞ 59 (Medium)

Turnover or dumpling—berry ☞ 59 (Medium)

Turnover or dumpling—cherry ☞ 59 (Medium)

Turnover or dumpling—lemon ☞ 59 (Medium)

Turnover or dumpling—peach ☞ 59 (Medium)

Turnover or dumpling—guava ☞ 59 (Medium)

Waffle—100% whole-wheat ☞ 76 (High)

Waffle—100% whole-grain ☞ 76 (High)

Waffle—fruit ☞ 76 (High)

Waffle—multi-bran ☞ 76 (High)

Waffle—nut and honey ☞ 76 (High)

Waffle—oat bran ☞ 76 (High)

Waffle—plain ☞ 76 (High)

Waffle—plain, fat free ☛ 76 (High)

Waffle—plain, lowfat ☛ 76 (High)

Waffle—multigrain ☛ 76 (High)

Waffle—bran ☛ 76 (High)

Waffle—wheat ☛ 76 (High)

16

CONDIMENTS, OILS & SAUCES

Beef Tallow ☛ 0 (Low)

Clarified Butter ☛ 0 (Low)

Cocktail sauce ☛ 38 (Low)

Dressing—Blue or roquefort ☛ 50 (Low)

Dressing—Blue or roquefort, low-calorie ☛ 50 (Low)

Dressing—Blue or roquefort, reduced calorie ☛ 50 (Low)

Dressing—Blue or roquefort, reduced calorie, fat-free ☛ 50 (Low)

Dressing—Caesar ☛ 50 (Low)

Dressing—Caesar, low-calorie ☛ 50 (Low)

Dressing—Coleslaw ☛ 50 (Low)

Dressing—Coleslaw, reduced calorie ☛ 50 (Low)

Dressing—Cream cheese ☛ 50 (Low)

Dressing—Creamy, prepared with sour cream, buttermilk and oil ☛ 50 (Low)

Dressing—Creamy, prepared with sour cream, diet ☞ 50 (Low)

Dressing—Creamy, prepared with sour cream, low calorie, cholesterol free ☞ 50 (Low)

Dressing—Creamy, prepared with sour cream, or buttermilk and oil ☞ 50 (Low)

Dressing—Creamy, prepared with sour cream, reduced calorie ☞ 50 (Low)

Dressing—Creamy, prepared with sour cream, reduced calorie, cholesterol-free ☞ 50 (Low)

Dressing—Feta Cheese ☞ 50 (Low)

Dressing—French ☞ 50 (Low)

Dressing—French, low calorie, fat free ☞ 50 (Low)

Dressing—French, reduced calorie ☞ 50 (Low)

Dressing—Green Goddess ☞ 50 (Low)

Dressing—Honey mustard ☞ 50 (Low)

Dressing—Italian dressing ☞ 50 (Low)

Dressing—Italian, diet or reduced calorie ☞ 50 (Low)

Dressing—Italian, diet or reduced calorie, fat free ☞ 50 (Low)

Dressing—Italian, reduced calorie ☞ 50 (Low)

Dressing—Korean ☞ 50 (Low)

Dressing—Mayonnaise-type salad, cholesterol-free ☞ 50 (Low)

Dressing—Mayonnaise-type salad, diet ☞ 50 (Low)

Dressing—Mayonnaise-type salad, fat-free ☞ 50 (Low)

Dressing—Mayonnaise-type salad, low calorie ☞ 50 (Low)

Dressing—Mayonnaise-type salad, Regular ☞ 50 (Low)

Dressing—Milk, vinegar based ☛ 50 (Low)

Dressing—Peppercorn ☛ 50 (Low)

Dressing—Poppy seed ☛ 50 (Low)

Dressing—Rice ☛ 64 (Low)

Dressing—Russian ☛ 50 (Low)

Dressing—Russian, low calorie ☛ 50 (Low)

Dressing—Salad dressing, low-calorie, without oil ☛ 50 (Low)

Dressing—Salad, common ☛ 50 (Low)

Dressing—Salad, low calorie ☛ 50 (Low)

Dressing—Sesame ☛ 50 (Low)

Dressing—Sweet and sour ☛ 50 (Low)

Dressing—Thousand Island Regular ☛ 50 (Low)

Dressing—Thousand Island, low-calorie ☛ 50 (Low)

Dressing—Thousand Island, reduced calorie, cholesterol free ☛ 50 (Low)

Dressing—Vinegar based ☛ 50 (Low)

Dressing—Yogurt ☛ 50 (Low)

Duck Fat ☛ 0 (Low)

French dressing, low-calorie ☛ 50 (Low)

Gravy—giblet ☛ 50 (Low)

Gravy—meat or poultry, with wine ☛ 50 (Low)

Gravy—meat, with fruit ☛ 50 (Low)

Gravy—mushroom ☛ 50 (Low)

Gravy—poultry ☛ 38 (Low)

Gravy—poultry, with wine ☞ 50 (Low)

Margarine ☞ 0 (Low)

Mayonnaise—diet or low-calorie ☞ 50 (Low)

Mayonnaise—diet or low-calorie, low sodium ☞ 50 (Low)

Mayonnaise—imitation ☞ 50 (Low)

Mayonnaise—low caloriet, cholesterol-free ☞ 50 (Low)

Mayonnaise—made with tofu ☞ 50 (Low)

Mayonnaise—made with yogurt ☞ 50 (Low)

Mayonnaise, regular ☞ 50 (Low)

Mustard greens—from canned, cooked, average value ☞ 32 (Low)

Mustard greens—from canned, cooked, with fat ☞ 32 (Low)

Mustard greens—from canned, cooked, without fat ☞ 32 (Low)

Mustard greens—from fresh, cooked, with fat ☞ 32 (Low)

Mustard greens—from fresh, cooked, without fat ☞ 32 (Low)

Mustard greens—from frozen, cooked, average value ☞ 32 (Low)

Mustard greens—from frozen, cooked, with fat ☞ 32 (Low)

Mustard greens—from frozen, cooked, without fat ☞ 32 (Low)

Mustard pickles ☞ 32 (Low)

Oil—Avocado ☞ 0 (Low)

Oil—Canola ☞ 0 (Low)

Oil—Coconut ☞ 0 (Low)

Oil—Corn ☞ 0 (Low)

Oil—Extra-virgin olive ☞ 0 (Low)

- Oil—Flaxseed ☛ 0 (Low)

- Oil—Grapeseed ☛ 0 (Low)

- Oil—Hazelnut ☛ 0 (Low)

- Oil—Hemp seed ☛ 0 (Low)

- Oil—Macadamia Nut ☛ 0 (Low)

- Oil—Olive ☛ 0 (Low)

- Oil—Palm ☛ 0 (Low)

- Oil—Peanut ☛ 0 (Low)

- Oil—Rice Bran ☛ 0 (Low)

- Oil—Safflower ☛ 0 (Low)

- Oil—Sesame ☛ 0 (Low)

- Oil—Soybean ☛ 0 (Low)

- Oil—Sunflower ☛ 0 (Low)

- Oil—Vegetable ☛ 0 (Low)

- Oil—Walnut ☛ 32 (Low)

- Sauce—Alfredo ☛ 27 (Low)

- Sauce—Cheese ☛ 27 (Low)

- Sauce—Cheese prepared with lowfat cheese ☛ 27 (Low)

- Sauce—Clam, white ☛ 27 (Low)

- Sauce—Tomato ☛ 38 (Low)

- Sauce—Tomato chili ☛ 38 (Low)

- Sauce—Tomato, low sodium ☛ 27 (Low)

- Sauce—White, or milk sauce ☛ 50 (Low)

Spaghetti sauce ☛ 38 (Low)

Spaghetti sauce—canned, with meat, canned ☛ 38 (Low)

Spaghetti sauce—homemade, fat free ☛ 38 (Low)

Spaghetti sauce—homemade, low salt ☛ 38 (Low)

Spaghetti sauce—homemade, with beef ☛ 38 (Low)

Spaghetti sauce—homemade, with combination of meats ☛ 38 (Low)

Spaghetti sauce—homemade, with lamb ☛ 38 (Low)

Spaghetti sauce—homemade, with meat ☛ 38 (Low)

Spaghetti sauce—homemade, with poultry ☛ 38 (Low)

Vinegar, sugar, and water dressing ☛ 0 (Low)

17

DAIRY FOODS & ALTERNATIVES

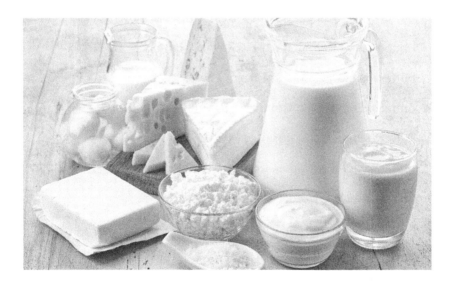

What is the serving size?

The typical serving sizes for low GI dairy products & oils are equivalent to:

- 1 cup of milk or yogurt

- ⅓ cup of cottage cheese
- 1 oz of cheese
- 1 teaspoon of oil or butter
- 1 teaspoon of margarine, or mayonnaise

For moderate GI Dairy Products & Alternatives reduce the serving by 1/3

How Much a Day?

Up to 3 servings per day

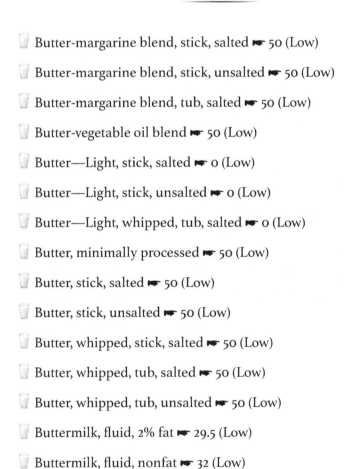

Butter-margarine blend, stick, salted ☛ 50 (Low)

Butter-margarine blend, stick, unsalted ☛ 50 (Low)

Butter-margarine blend, tub, salted ☛ 50 (Low)

Butter-vegetable oil blend ☛ 50 (Low)

Butter—Light, stick, salted ☛ 0 (Low)

Butter—Light, stick, unsalted ☛ 0 (Low)

Butter—Light, whipped, tub, salted ☛ 0 (Low)

Butter, minimally processed ☛ 50 (Low)

Butter, stick, salted ☛ 50 (Low)

Butter, stick, unsalted ☛ 50 (Low)

Butter, whipped, stick, salted ☛ 50 (Low)

Butter, whipped, tub, salted ☛ 50 (Low)

Butter, whipped, tub, unsalted ☛ 50 (Low)

Buttermilk, fluid, 2% fat ☛ 29.5 (Low)

Buttermilk, fluid, nonfat ☛ 32 (Low)

Carry-out milk shake, chocolate ☞ 44 (Low)

Carry-out milk shake, flavors other than chocolate ☞ 44 (Low)

Cheese—Amercican style ☞ 27 (Low)

Cheese—Blue ☞ 0.0 (Low)

Cheese—camembert ☞ 25 (Low)

Cheese—cheddar ☞ 27 (Low)

Cheese—Colby ☞ 27 (Low)

Cheese—cottage, low-fat ☞ 10 (Low)

Cheese—cottage, minimally processed ☞ 29.5 (Low)

Cheese—cottage, reduced-fat ☞ 10 (Low)

Cheese—cottage, regular-fat ☞ 10 (Low)

Cheese—cottage, salted, dry curd ☞ 32 (Low)

Cheese—cottage, with fruit ☞ 42.5 (Low)

Cheese—cream ☞ 27 (Low)

Cheese—cream, lowfat ☞ 27 (Low)

Cheese—Edam ☞ 27 (Low)

Cheese—Feta ☞ 27 (Low)

Cheese—Fontina ☞ 27 (Low)

Cheese—goat ☞ 27 (Low)

Cheese—Gouda ☞ 27 (Low)

Cheese—Gruyere ☞ 27 (Low)

Cheese—halloumi ☞ 0.0 (Low)

Cheese—havarti ☞ 0.0 (Low)

Cheese—Limburger ☛ 27 (Low)

Cheese—Manchego ☛ 27 (Low)

Cheese—Monterey ☛ 27 (Low)

Cheese—mozzarella ☛ 27 (Low)

Cheese—Mozzarella, low sodium ☛ 27 (Low)

Cheese—Mozzarella, average value ☛ 27 (Low)

Cheese—Mozzarella, nonfat or fat free ☛ 32 (Low)

Cheese—Mozzarella, part skim ☛ 27 (Low)

Cheese—Muenster ☛ 27 (Low)

Cheese—Muenster, lowfat ☛ 27 (Low)

Cheese—natural, Cheddar or American type ☛ 27 (Low)

Cheese—natural, minimally processed ☛ 27 (Low)

Cheese—minimally processed ☛ 27 (Low)

Cheese—Parmesan ☛ 27 (Low)

Cheese—Parmesan, dry grated ☛ 27 (Low)

Cheese—Parmesan, hard ☛ 27 (Low)

Cheese—Parmesan, low sodium ☛ 27 (Low)

Cheese—Pecorino Romano ☛ 0.0 (Low)

Cheese—processed cheese common ☛ 27 (Low)

Cheese—processed cheese, American type based ☛ 27 (Low)

Cheese—processed cheese, Cheddar based ☛ 27 (Low)

Cheese—processed cheese, Swiss based ☛ 27 (Low)

Cheese—processed cream cheese ☛ 32 (Low)

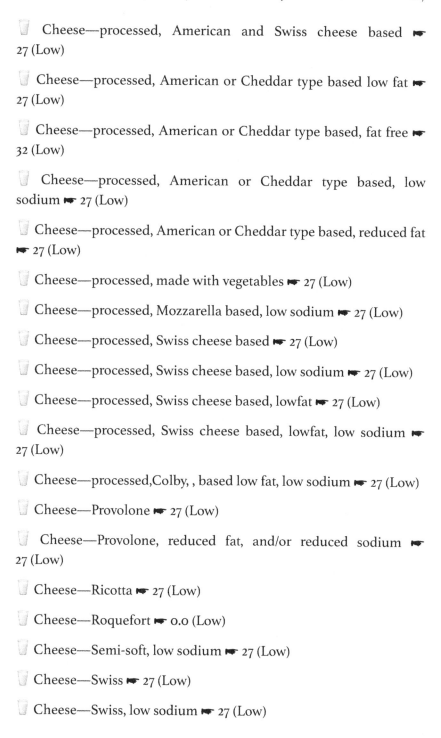

Cheese—processed, American and Swiss cheese based ☞ 27 (Low)

Cheese—processed, American or Cheddar type based low fat ☞ 27 (Low)

Cheese—processed, American or Cheddar type based, fat free ☞ 32 (Low)

Cheese—processed, American or Cheddar type based, low sodium ☞ 27 (Low)

Cheese—processed, American or Cheddar type based, reduced fat ☞ 27 (Low)

Cheese—processed, made with vegetables ☞ 27 (Low)

Cheese—processed, Mozzarella based, low sodium ☞ 27 (Low)

Cheese—processed, Swiss cheese based ☞ 27 (Low)

Cheese—processed, Swiss cheese based, low sodium ☞ 27 (Low)

Cheese—processed, Swiss cheese based, lowfat ☞ 27 (Low)

Cheese—processed, Swiss cheese based, lowfat, low sodium ☞ 27 (Low)

Cheese—processed,Colby, , based low fat, low sodium ☞ 27 (Low)

Cheese—Provolone ☞ 27 (Low)

Cheese—Provolone, reduced fat, and/or reduced sodium ☞ 27 (Low)

Cheese—Ricotta ☞ 27 (Low)

Cheese—Roquefort ☞ 0.0 (Low)

Cheese—Semi-soft, low sodium ☞ 27 (Low)

Cheese—Swiss ☞ 27 (Low)

Cheese—Swiss, low sodium ☞ 27 (Low)

- Cheese—Swiss, lowfat ☛ 27 (Low)
- Cheese—yogurt, common ☛ 27 (Low)
- Cow's—Milk skim ☛ 40 (Low)
- Cow's—Milk full cream ☛ 40 (Low)
- Cow's—Milk reduced fat ☛ 40 (Low)
- Cream cheese ☛ 0.0 (Low)
- Cream substitute—frozen ☛ 27 (Low)
- Cream substitute—frozen, liquid, and/or powdered ☛ 27 (Low)
- Cream substitute—light, liquid ☛ 27 (Low)
- Cream substitute—light, powdered ☛ 27 (Low)
- Cream substitute—liquid ☛ 27 (Low)
- Cream substitute—powdered ☛ 27 (Low)
- Cream—average value, half and half ☛ 27 (Low)
- Cream—half and half ☛ 27 (Low)
- Cream—heavy, fluid ☛ 27 (Low)
- Cream—heavy, whipped and lightly sweetened ☛ 55.4 (Medium)
- Cream—light, fluid ☛ 27 (Low)
- Cream—light, whipped, and unsweetened ☛ 27 (Low)
- Cream—pure regular-fat ☛ 0.0 (Low)
- Cream—sour ☛ 0.0 (Low)
- Cream—thickened regular-fat ☛ 0.0 (Low)
- Cream—whipped ☛ 0.0 (Low)
- Cream—whipped, purchased as pressurized container ☛ 55.4 (Medium)

Custard homemade ☛ 29 (Low)

Custard industrially made ☛ 38 (Low)

Custard—Puerto Rican style ☛ 38 (Low)

Dip—cream cheese base ☛ 27 (Low)

Dip—sour cream base ☛ 27 (Low)

Dip—sour cream base, low calorie ☛ 27 (Low)

Dip, cheese—chili con queso ☛ 27 (Low)

Ghee ☛ 0.0 (Low)

Goat—Cheese ☛ 27 (Low)

Goat—Cheese plain ☛ 0.0 (Low)

Goat's—Milk whole ☛ 40 (Low)

Goat's—milk yoghurt ☛ 25 (Low)

Ice cream—average value ☛ 61 (Medium)

Ice cream—bar or stick, not covered by chocolate ☛ 61 (Medium)

Ice cream—regular, chocolate ☛ 61 (Medium)

Ice cream—regular, flavors other than chocolate ☛ 61 (Medium)

Ice cream—rich, chocolate ☛ 37 (Low)

Ice cream—rich, flavors other than chocolate ☛ 38 (Low)

Ice cream—soda, chocolate ☛ 59.5 (Medium)

Ice cream—soda, flavors other than chocolate ☛ 64.5 (Medium)

Ice cream—soft serve, average value ☛ 61 (Medium)

Ice cream—soft serve, chocolate ☛ 61 (Medium)

Ice cream—soft serve, flavors other than chocolate ☛ 61 (Medium)

Ice cream—with sherbet ☞ 51.5 (Low)

Ice-cream ☞ 63 (Medium)

Imitation cheese—American type ☞ 27 (Low)

Imitation cheese—cheddar ☞ 27 (Low)

Imitation cheese—Edam ☞ 27 (Low)

Imitation cheese—Mozzarella ☞ 27 (Low)

Kefir ☞ 32 (Low)

Light ice cream—chocolate ☞ 50 (Low)

Light ice cream—flavors other than chocolate ☞ 50 (Low)

Light ice cream—fudgesicle ☞ 50 (Low)

Light ice cream—NFS ☞ 50 (Low)

Light ice cream—premium, chocolate ☞ 50 (Low)

Light ice cream—premium, flavors other than chocolate ☞ 50 (Low)

Light ice cream—soft serve, chocolate ☞ 50 (Low)

Light ice cream—soft serve, flavors other than chocolate ☞ 50 (Low)

Light ice cream—soft serve, NS as to flavor ☞ 50 (Low)

Light ice cream—with sherbet ☞ 46 (Low)

Margarine-based spread—fat free, liquid, salted ☞ 50 (Low)

Margarine-based spread—fat free, tub, salted ☞ 50 (Low)

Margarine-based spread—liquid, salted ☞ 0 (Low)

Margarine-based spread—reduced calorie, about 20% fat, tub, salted ☞ 0 (Low)

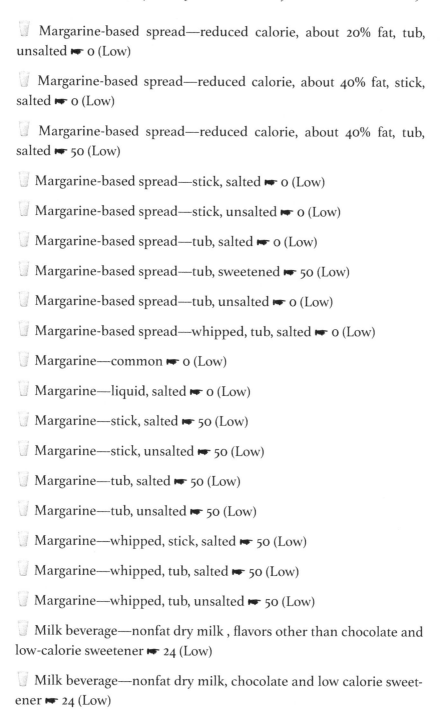

Margarine-based spread—reduced calorie, about 20% fat, tub, unsalted ☞ 0 (Low)

Margarine-based spread—reduced calorie, about 40% fat, stick, salted ☞ 0 (Low)

Margarine-based spread—reduced calorie, about 40% fat, tub, salted ☞ 50 (Low)

Margarine-based spread—stick, salted ☞ 0 (Low)

Margarine-based spread—stick, unsalted ☞ 0 (Low)

Margarine-based spread—tub, salted ☞ 0 (Low)

Margarine-based spread—tub, sweetened ☞ 50 (Low)

Margarine-based spread—tub, unsalted ☞ 0 (Low)

Margarine-based spread—whipped, tub, salted ☞ 0 (Low)

Margarine—common ☞ 0 (Low)

Margarine—liquid, salted ☞ 0 (Low)

Margarine—stick, salted ☞ 50 (Low)

Margarine—stick, unsalted ☞ 50 (Low)

Margarine—tub, salted ☞ 50 (Low)

Margarine—tub, unsalted ☞ 50 (Low)

Margarine—whipped, stick, salted ☞ 50 (Low)

Margarine—whipped, tub, salted ☞ 50 (Low)

Margarine—whipped, tub, unsalted ☞ 50 (Low)

Milk beverage—nonfat dry milk , flavors other than chocolate and low-calorie sweetener ☞ 24 (Low)

Milk beverage—nonfat dry milk, chocolate and low calorie sweetener ☞ 24 (Low)

Milk beverage—whole milk, flavors other than chocolate ☞ 35 (Low)

Milk dessert—frozen, chocolate (no butterfat) ☞ 61 (Medium)

Milk dessert—frozen, chocolate ☞ 61 (Medium)

Milk dessert—frozen, flavors other than chocolate ☞ 61 (Medium)

Milk dessert—frozen, flavors other than chocolate ☞ 61 (Medium)

Milk dessert—frozen, flavors other than chocolate, low calorie sweetener ☞ 50 (Low)

Milk dessert—frozen, flavors other than chocolate, lowfat ☞ 50 (Low)

Milk dessert—frozen, low-calorie sweetener ☞ 50 (Low)

Milk dessert—frozen, lowfat, flavors other than chocolate ☞ 50 (Low)

Milk gravy ☞ 50 (Low)

Milk lactose—free ☞ 40 (Low)

Milk made from soy protein ☞ 50 (Low)

Milk shake—average value ☞ 44 (Low)

Milk shake—common ☞ 44 (Low)

Milk shake—homemade, chocolate ☞ 44 (Low)

Milk shake—homemade, chocolate ☞ 44 (Low)

Milk shake—homemade, flavors other than chocolate ☞ 44 (Low)

Milk shake—homemade, flavors other than chocolate ☞ 44 (Low)

Milk shake—made with skim milk, chocolate ☞ 46.5 (Low)

Milk shake—made with skim milk, flavors other than chocolate ☞ 46.5 (Low)

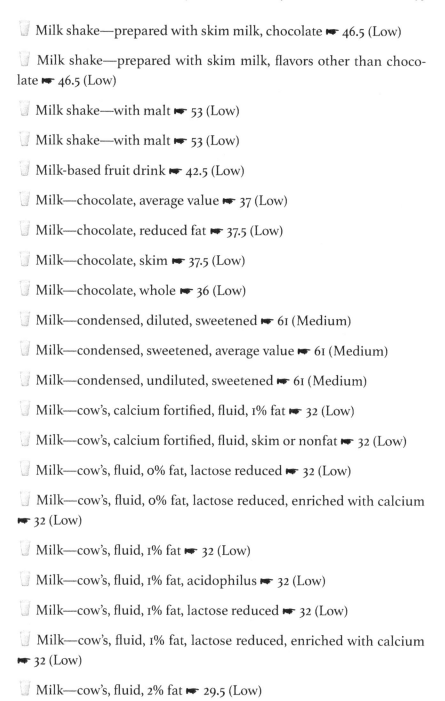

Milk shake—prepared with skim milk, chocolate ☛ 46.5 (Low)

Milk shake—prepared with skim milk, flavors other than chocolate ☛ 46.5 (Low)

Milk shake—with malt ☛ 53 (Low)

Milk shake—with malt ☛ 53 (Low)

Milk-based fruit drink ☛ 42.5 (Low)

Milk—chocolate, average value ☛ 37 (Low)

Milk—chocolate, reduced fat ☛ 37.5 (Low)

Milk—chocolate, skim ☛ 37.5 (Low)

Milk—chocolate, whole ☛ 36 (Low)

Milk—condensed, diluted, sweetened ☛ 61 (Medium)

Milk—condensed, sweetened, average value ☛ 61 (Medium)

Milk—condensed, undiluted, sweetened ☛ 61 (Medium)

Milk—cow's, calcium fortified, fluid, 1% fat ☛ 32 (Low)

Milk—cow's, calcium fortified, fluid, skim or nonfat ☛ 32 (Low)

Milk—cow's, fluid, 0% fat, lactose reduced ☛ 32 (Low)

Milk—cow's, fluid, 0% fat, lactose reduced, enriched with calcium ☛ 32 (Low)

Milk—cow's, fluid, 1% fat ☛ 32 (Low)

Milk—cow's, fluid, 1% fat, acidophilus ☛ 32 (Low)

Milk—cow's, fluid, 1% fat, lactose reduced ☛ 32 (Low)

Milk—cow's, fluid, 1% fat, lactose reduced, enriched with calcium ☛ 32 (Low)

Milk—cow's, fluid, 2% fat ☛ 29.5 (Low)

Milk—cow's, fluid, 2% fat, acidophilus ☞ 29.5 (Low)

Milk—cow's, fluid, 2% fat, lactose reduced ☞ 29.5 (Low)

Milk—cow's, fluid, whole ☞ 27 (Low)

Milk—dry, reconstituted, 0% fat ☞ 32 (Low)

Milk—dry, reconstituted, average value ☞ 32 (Low)

Milk—dry, reconstituted, lowfat ☞ 32 (Low)

Milk—dry, reconstituted, whole ☞ 27 (Low)

Milk—evaporated ☞ 40 (Low)

Milk—evaporated, undiluted ☞ 27 (Low)

Milk—evaporated, 2% fat, dilution not specified ☞ 27 (Low)

Milk—evaporated, 2% fat, undiluted ☞ 27 (Low)

Milk—evaporated, average value for fat content and dilution ☞ 27 (Low)

Milk—evaporated, skim, undiluted ☞ 32 (Low)

Milk—evaporated, skim, used in coffee or tea ☞ 32 (Low)

Milk—evaporated, used in coffee or tea ☞ 27 (Low)

Milk—evaporated, whole, diluted ☞ 27 (Low)

Milk—evaporated, whole, NS as to dilution ☞ 27 (Low)

Milk—evaporated, whole, undiluted ☞ 27 (Low)

Milk—evaporated, whole, used in coffee or tea ☞ 27 (Low)

Milk—flavors other than chocolate, whole milk-based ☞ 35 (Low)

Milk—goat's, fluid, whole ☞ 27 (Low)

Milk—imitation, fluid, soy based ☞ 40 (Low)

Milk—malted, fortified, chocolate, made with milk ☞ 45 (Low)

Milk—malted, fortified, natural flavor, made with milk ☛ 45 (Low)

Milk—malted, fortified, NS as to flavor, made with milk ☛ 45 (Low)

Milk—malted, unfortified, NS as to flavor, made with milk ☛ 45 (Low)

Milk—NFS ☛ 29.5 (Low)

Milk—soy, dry, reconstituted, not baby's ☛ 40 (Low)

Milk—soy, ready-to-drink, not baby's ☛ 40 (Low)

Milk—vinegar, and sugar dressing ☛ 50 (Low)

Milk—whole ☛ 40 (Low)

Milk, almond ☛ 25 (Low)

Milk, coconut ☛ 41 (Low)

Milk, hemp ☛ 0.0 (Low)

Milk, oat ☛ 105 (High)

Milk, rice ☛ 86 (High)

Milk, soy, beans ☛ 41 (Low)

Mousse—chocolate ☛ 34 (Low)

Mousse—not chocolate ☛ 34 (Low)

Oatmilk ☛ 105 (High)

Pudding—canned, chocolate ☛ 44 (Low)

Pudding—canned, chocolate and non-chocolate flavors combined ☛ 44 (Low)

Pudding—canned, chocolate, fat free ☛ 44 (Low)

Pudding—canned, chocolate, reduced fat ☛ 44 (Low)

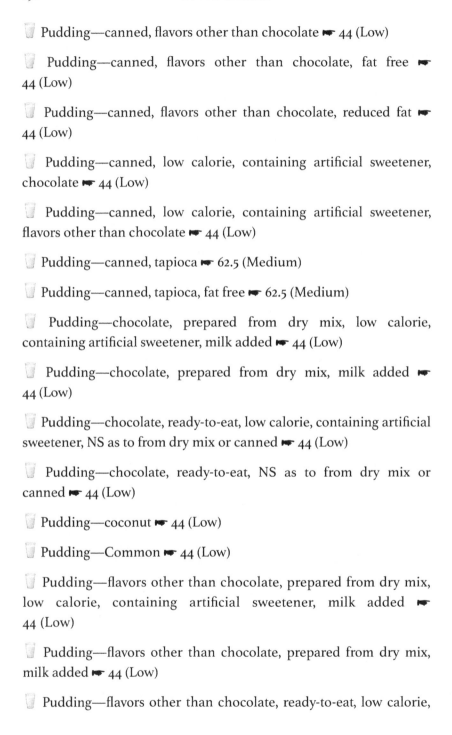

Pudding—canned, flavors other than chocolate ☞ 44 (Low)

Pudding—canned, flavors other than chocolate, fat free ☞ 44 (Low)

Pudding—canned, flavors other than chocolate, reduced fat ☞ 44 (Low)

Pudding—canned, low calorie, containing artificial sweetener, chocolate ☞ 44 (Low)

Pudding—canned, low calorie, containing artificial sweetener, flavors other than chocolate ☞ 44 (Low)

Pudding—canned, tapioca ☞ 62.5 (Medium)

Pudding—canned, tapioca, fat free ☞ 62.5 (Medium)

Pudding—chocolate, prepared from dry mix, low calorie, containing artificial sweetener, milk added ☞ 44 (Low)

Pudding—chocolate, prepared from dry mix, milk added ☞ 44 (Low)

Pudding—chocolate, ready-to-eat, low calorie, containing artificial sweetener, NS as to from dry mix or canned ☞ 44 (Low)

Pudding—chocolate, ready-to-eat, NS as to from dry mix or canned ☞ 44 (Low)

Pudding—coconut ☞ 44 (Low)

Pudding—Common ☞ 44 (Low)

Pudding—flavors other than chocolate, prepared from dry mix, low calorie, containing artificial sweetener, milk added ☞ 44 (Low)

Pudding—flavors other than chocolate, prepared from dry mix, milk added ☞ 44 (Low)

Pudding—flavors other than chocolate, ready-to-eat, low calorie, containing artificial sweetener, NS as to from dry mix or canned 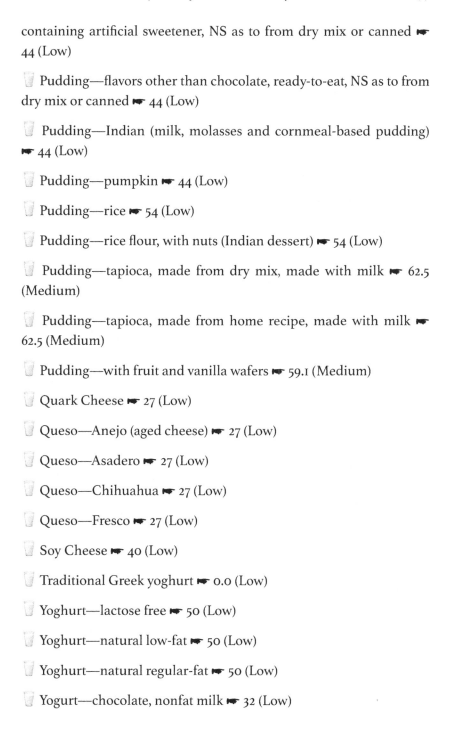 44 (Low)

Pudding—flavors other than chocolate, ready-to-eat, NS as to from dry mix or canned 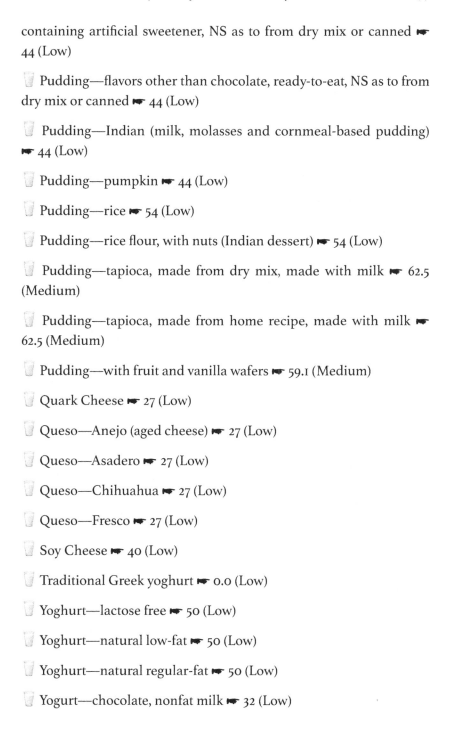 44 (Low)

Pudding—Indian (milk, molasses and cornmeal-based pudding) 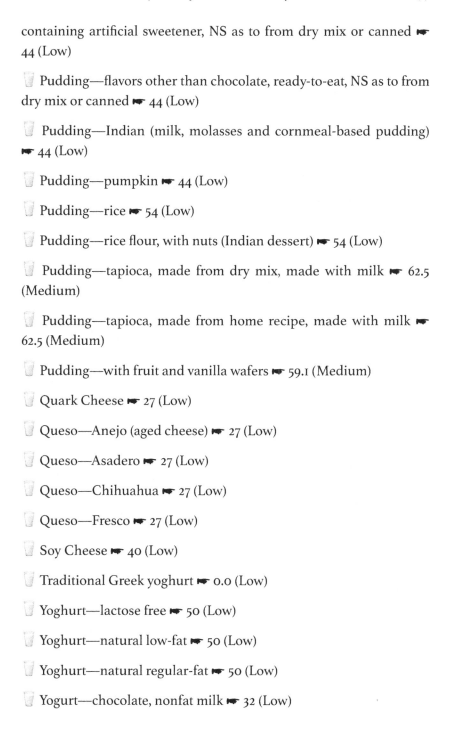 44 (Low)

Pudding—pumpkin 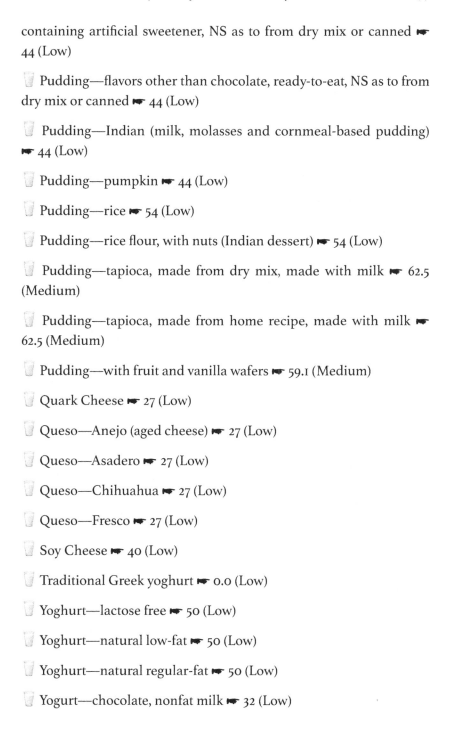 44 (Low)

Pudding—rice 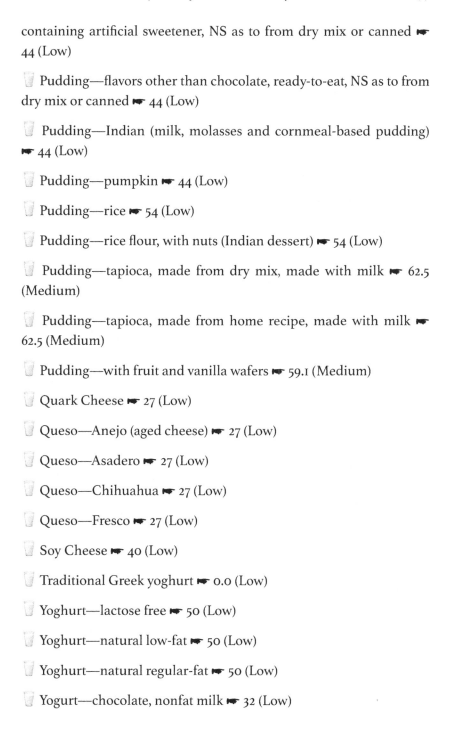 54 (Low)

Pudding—rice flour, with nuts (Indian dessert) 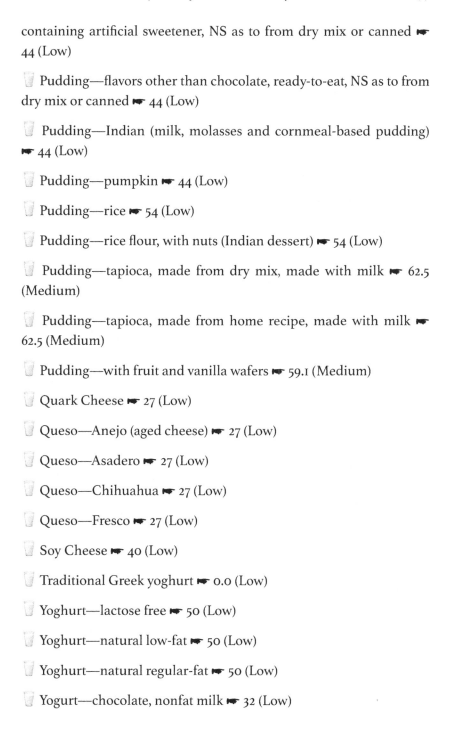 54 (Low)

Pudding—tapioca, made from dry mix, made with milk 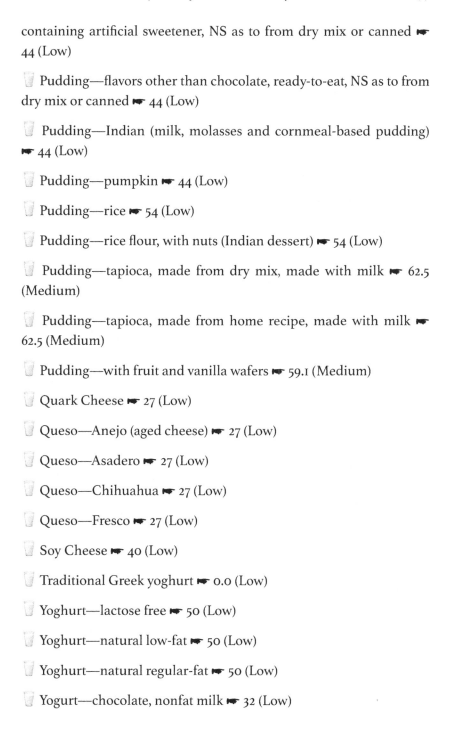 62.5 (Medium)

Pudding—tapioca, made from home recipe, made with milk 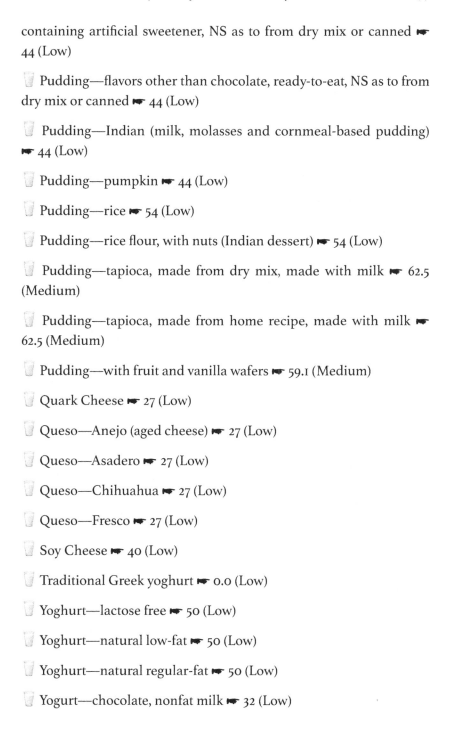 62.5 (Medium)

Pudding—with fruit and vanilla wafers 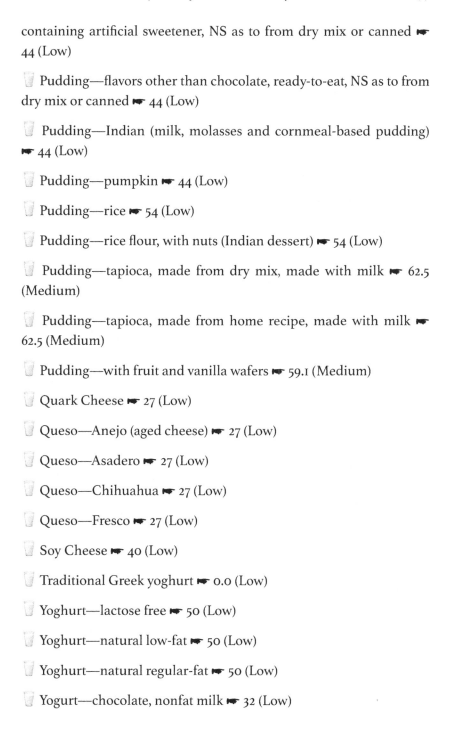 59.1 (Medium)

Quark Cheese 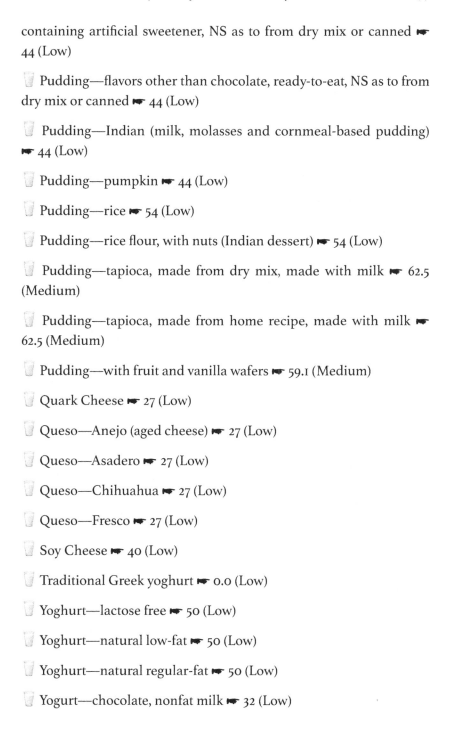 27 (Low)

Queso—Anejo (aged cheese) 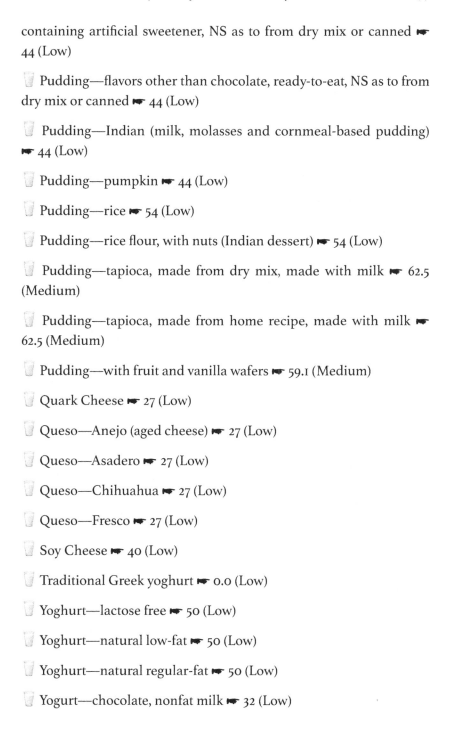 27 (Low)

Queso—Asadero 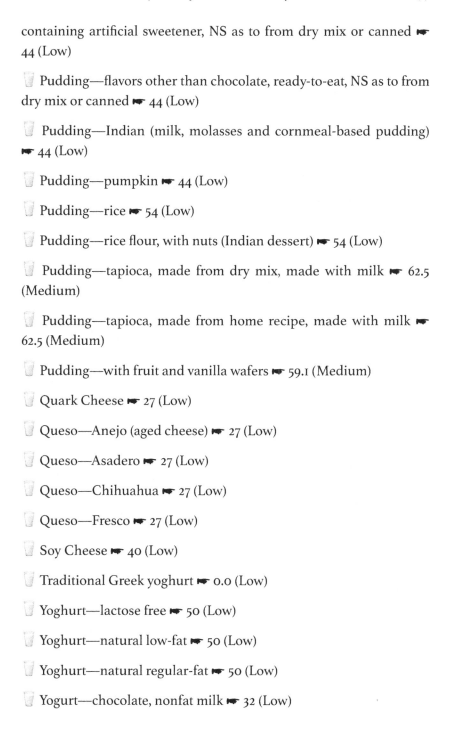 27 (Low)

Queso—Chihuahua 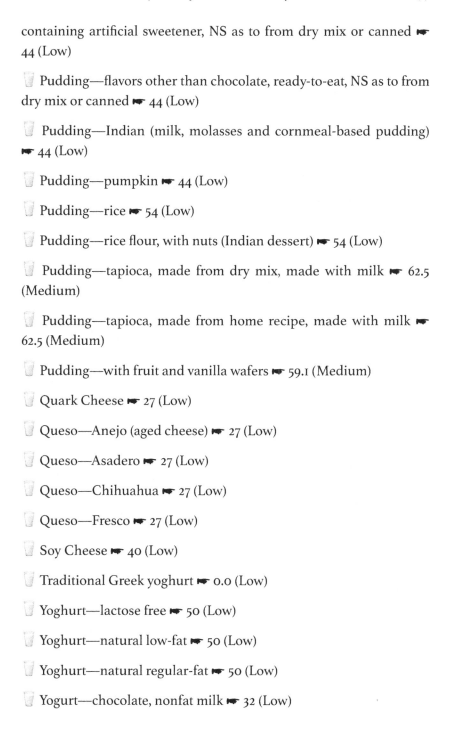 27 (Low)

Queso—Fresco 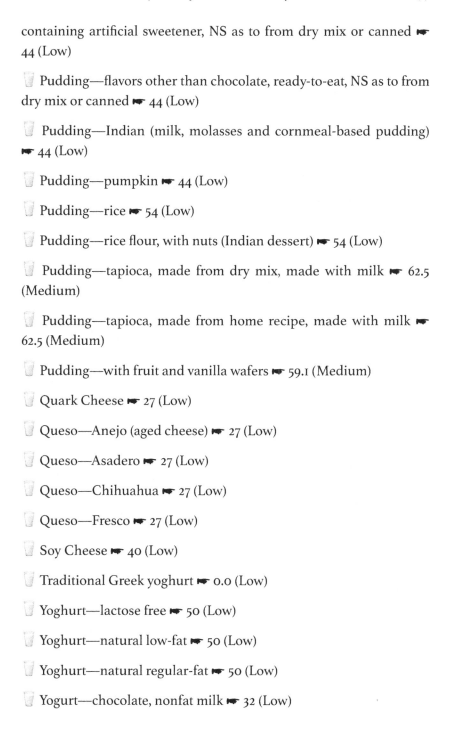 27 (Low)

Soy Cheese 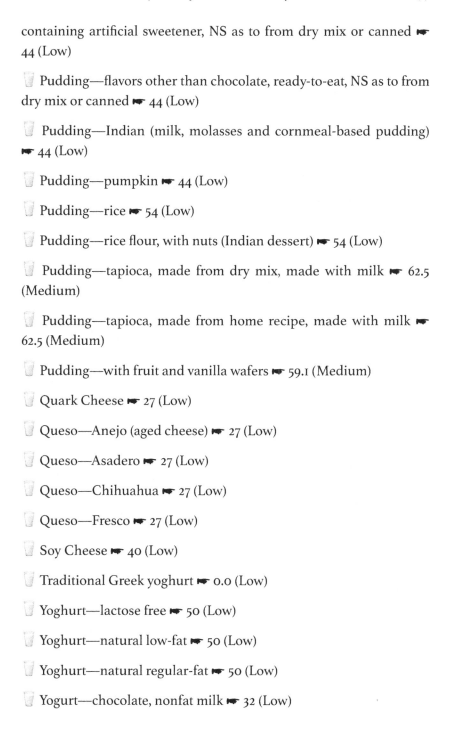 40 (Low)

Traditional Greek yoghurt 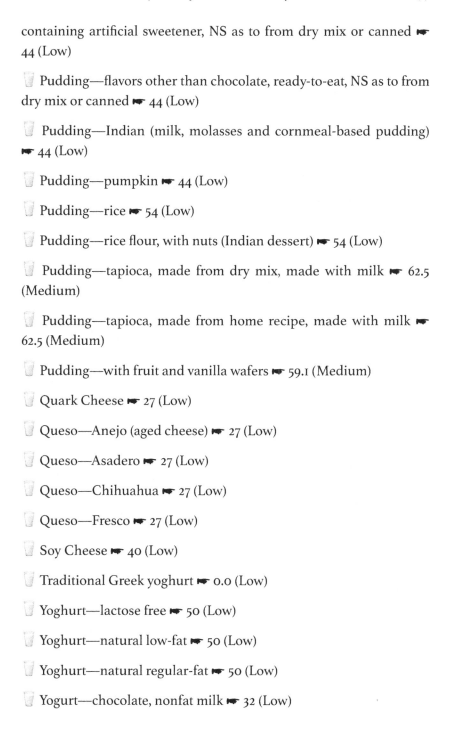 0.0 (Low)

Yoghurt—lactose free 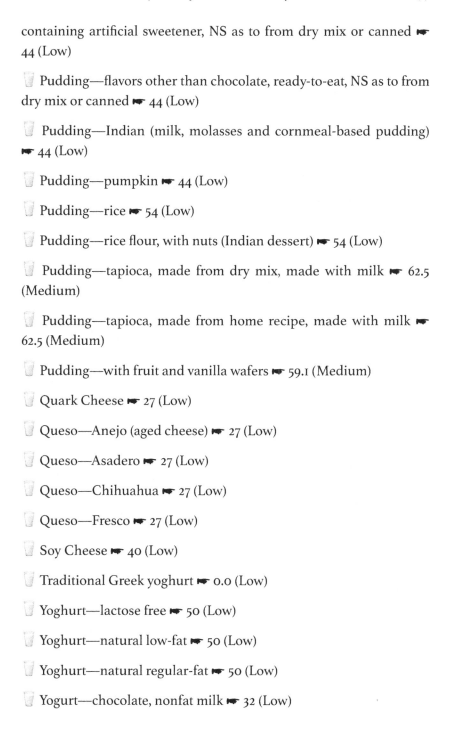 50 (Low)

Yoghurt—natural low-fat 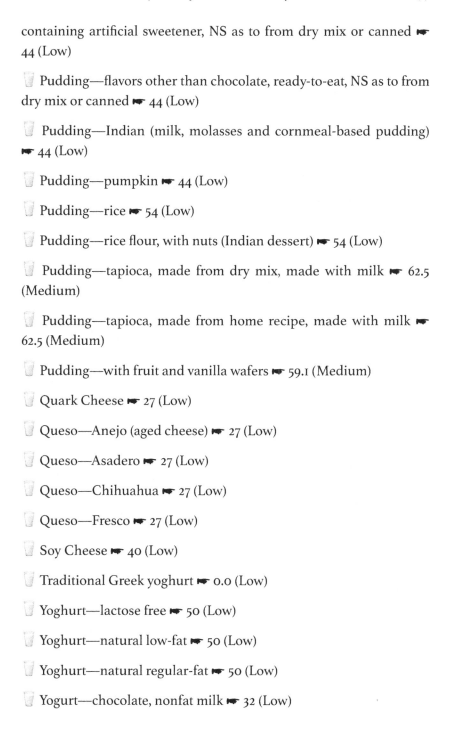 50 (Low)

Yoghurt—natural regular-fat 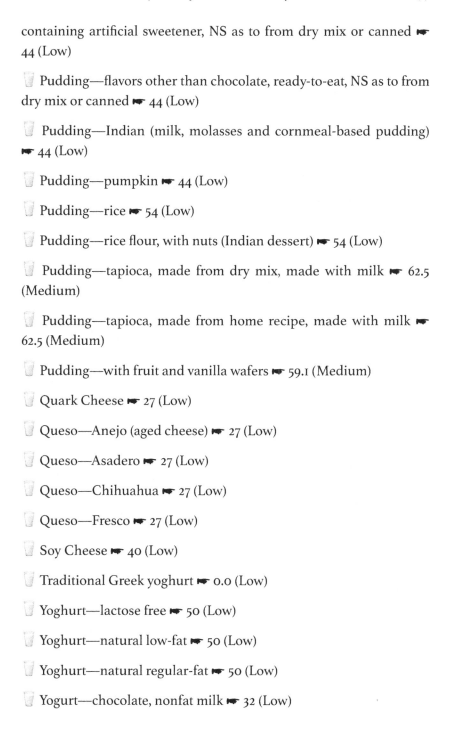 50 (Low)

Yogurt—chocolate, nonfat milk 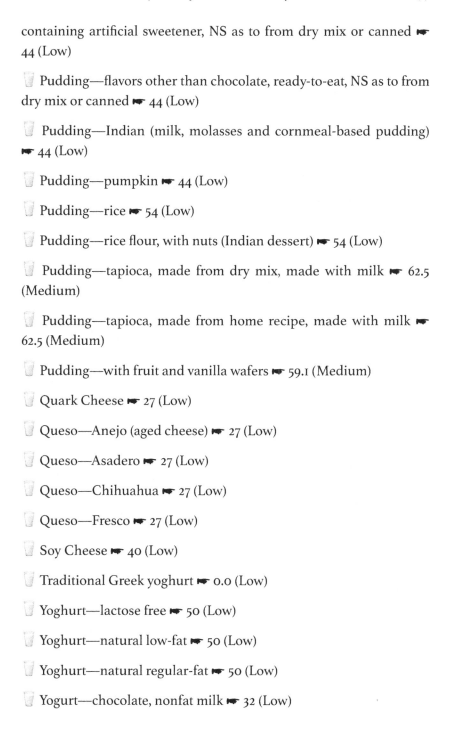 32 (Low)

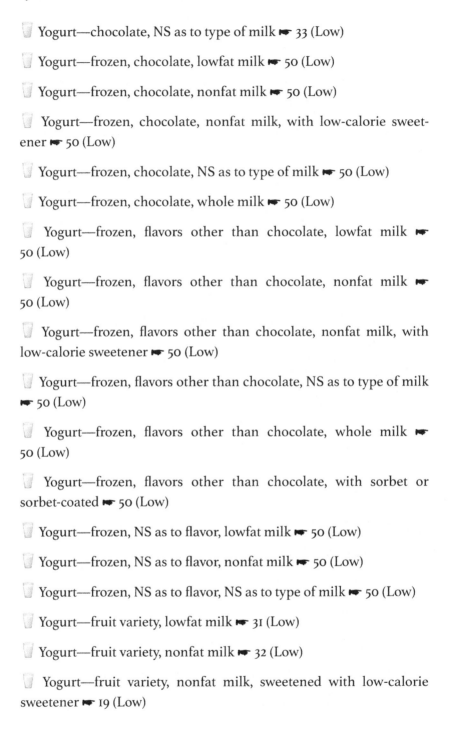

Yogurt—chocolate, NS as to type of milk ☞ 33 (Low)

Yogurt—frozen, chocolate, lowfat milk ☞ 50 (Low)

Yogurt—frozen, chocolate, nonfat milk ☞ 50 (Low)

Yogurt—frozen, chocolate, nonfat milk, with low-calorie sweetener ☞ 50 (Low)

Yogurt—frozen, chocolate, NS as to type of milk ☞ 50 (Low)

Yogurt—frozen, chocolate, whole milk ☞ 50 (Low)

Yogurt—frozen, flavors other than chocolate, lowfat milk ☞ 50 (Low)

Yogurt—frozen, flavors other than chocolate, nonfat milk ☞ 50 (Low)

Yogurt—frozen, flavors other than chocolate, nonfat milk, with low-calorie sweetener ☞ 50 (Low)

Yogurt—frozen, flavors other than chocolate, NS as to type of milk ☞ 50 (Low)

Yogurt—frozen, flavors other than chocolate, whole milk ☞ 50 (Low)

Yogurt—frozen, flavors other than chocolate, with sorbet or sorbet-coated ☞ 50 (Low)

Yogurt—frozen, NS as to flavor, lowfat milk ☞ 50 (Low)

Yogurt—frozen, NS as to flavor, nonfat milk ☞ 50 (Low)

Yogurt—frozen, NS as to flavor, NS as to type of milk ☞ 50 (Low)

Yogurt—fruit variety, lowfat milk ☞ 31 (Low)

Yogurt—fruit variety, nonfat milk ☞ 32 (Low)

Yogurt—fruit variety, nonfat milk, sweetened with low-calorie sweetener ☞ 19 (Low)

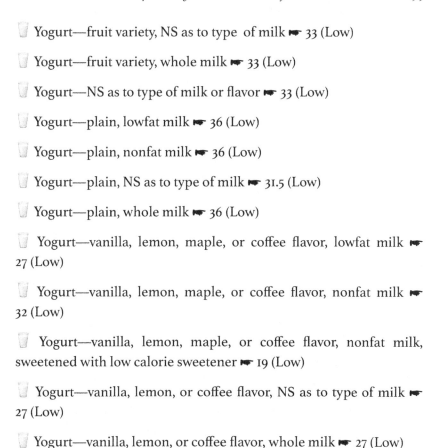

Yogurt—fruit variety, NS as to type of milk ☛ 33 (Low)

Yogurt—fruit variety, whole milk ☛ 33 (Low)

Yogurt—NS as to type of milk or flavor ☛ 33 (Low)

Yogurt—plain, lowfat milk ☛ 36 (Low)

Yogurt—plain, nonfat milk ☛ 36 (Low)

Yogurt—plain, NS as to type of milk ☛ 31.5 (Low)

Yogurt—plain, whole milk ☛ 36 (Low)

Yogurt—vanilla, lemon, maple, or coffee flavor, lowfat milk ☛ 27 (Low)

Yogurt—vanilla, lemon, maple, or coffee flavor, nonfat milk ☛ 32 (Low)

Yogurt—vanilla, lemon, maple, or coffee flavor, nonfat milk, sweetened with low calorie sweetener ☛ 19 (Low)

Yogurt—vanilla, lemon, or coffee flavor, NS as to type of milk ☛ 27 (Low)

Yogurt—vanilla, lemon, or coffee flavor, whole milk ☛ 27 (Low)

18

FISH & FISH PRODUCTS

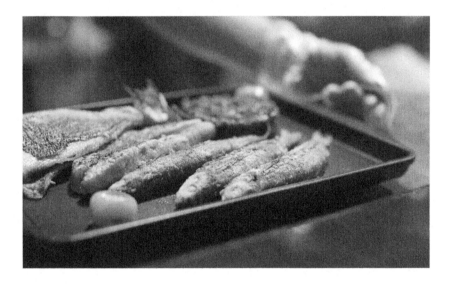

What is the serving size?

The typical serving sizes for low GI Fishes & Fishes Products are equivalent to:

- 3 to 4 ounces of cooked or canned fish
- 3 to 4 ounces of seafood

For moderate GI Fish & Fish Products reduce the serving by 1/3

How Much a Day?

Up to 3 servings per day

Anchovy—canned, oil or water ☞ 0 (Low)

Anchovy—cooked, average value for cooking method ☞ 0 (Low)

Carp—baked or broiled ☞ 50 (Low)

Carp—floured or breaded, fried ☞ 95 (High)

Carp—steamed or poached ☞ 0 (Low)

Catfish—baked or broiled ☞ 50 (Low)

Catfish—battered, fried ☞ 95 (High)

Catfish—breaded or battered, baked ☞ 95 (High)

Catfish—floured or breaded, fried ☞ 95 (High)

Catfish—steamed or poached ☞ 0 (Low)

Clams—baked or broiled ☞ 50 (Low)

Clams—battered, fried ☞ 95 (High)

Clams—canned, oil or water ☞ 50 (Low)

Clams—floured or breaded, fried ☞ 95 (High)

Clams—raw ☞ 50 (Low)

Clams—steamed or boiled ☞ 50 (Low)

🐸 Cod—baked or broiled ☛ 50 (Low)

🐸 Cod—battered, fried ☛ 95 (High)

🐸 Cod—breaded or battered, baked ☛ 95 (High)

🐸 Cod—floured or breaded, fried ☛ 95 (High)

🐸 Cod—steamed or poached ☛ 0 (Low)

🐸 Conch—baked or broiled ☛ 50 (Low)

🐸 Crab—baked or broiled ☛ 50 (Low)

🐸 Crab—cooked, average for the cooking method ☛ 0 (Low)

🐸 Crab—hard shell, steamed ☛ 0 (Low)

🐸 Crab—soft shell, floured, fried ☛ 95 (High)

🐸 Crayfish—floured, fried ☛ 95 (High)

🐸 Croaker—baked or broiled ☛ 50 (Low)

🐸 Croaker—floured or breaded, fried ☛ 95 (High)

🐸 Croaker—steamed or poached ☛ 0 (Low)

🐸 Eel—cooked, average value for cooking method ☛ 95 (High)

🐸 Fish stick—patty, or fillet ☛ 95 (High)

🐸 Fish stick—patty, or fillet, baked or broiled ☛ 95 (High)

🐸 Fish stick—patty, or fillet, battered, fried ☛ 95 (High)

🐸 Fish stick—patty, or fillet, breaded or battered, baked ☛ 95 (High)

🐸 Fish stick—patty, or fillet, NS as to type—floured or breaded, fried ☛ 95 (High)

🐸 Fish, in general—baked or broiled ☛ 50 (Low)

🐸 Fish, in general—battered, fried ☛ 95 (High)

Fish, in general—breaded or battered, baked ☞ 95 (High)

Fish, in general—canned ☞ 0 (Low)

Fish, in general—floured or breaded, fried ☞ 95 (High)

Fish, in general—smoked ☞ 0 (Low)

Fish, in general—steamed ☞ 0 (Low)

Flounder—baked or broiled ☞ 50 (Low)

Flounder—battered, fried ☞ 95 (High)

Flounder—breaded or battered, baked ☞ 95 (High)

Flounder—cooked, average value for cooking method ☞ 50 (Low)

Flounder—floured or breaded, fried ☞ 95 (High)

Flounder—steamed or poached ☞ 0 (Low)

Haddock—baked or broiled ☞ 50 (Low)

Haddock—battered, fried ☞ 95 (High)

Haddock—breaded or battered, baked ☞ 95 (High)

Haddock—floured or breaded, fried ☞ 95 (High)

Haddock—steamed or poached ☞ 0 (Low)

Haddock, cooked, average value for cooking method ☞ 50 (Low)

Herring—baked or broiled ☞ 50 (Low)

Herring—pickled ☞ 50 (Low)

Herring—raw ☞ 0 (Low)

Herring—smoked, kippered ☞ 0 (Low)

Lobster—baked or broiled ☞ 50 (Low)

Lobster—cooked, average value for cooking method ☞ 50 (Low)

🦞 Lobster—steamed or boiled ☞ 50 (Low)

🦞 Lobster—without shell, steamed or boiled ☞ 50 (Low)

🦞 Mackerel—baked or broiled ☞ 50 (Low)

🦞 Mackerel—canned ☞ 0 (Low)

🦞 Mackerel—cooked, average value for cooking method ☞ 50 (Low)

🦞 Mackerel—floured or breaded, fried ☞ 95 (High)

🦞 Mullet—baked or broiled ☞ 50 (Low)

🦞 Mullet—floured or breaded, fried ☞ 95 (High)

🦞 Mussels—cooked, average value for cooking method ☞ 95 (High)

🦞 Mussels—steamed or poached ☞ 50 (Low)

🦞 Ocean perch—baked or broiled ☞ 50 (Low)

🦞 Ocean perch—battered, fried ☞ 95 (High)

🦞 Ocean perch—breaded or battered, baked ☞ 95 (High)

🦞 Ocean perch—floured or breaded, fried ☞ 95 (High)

🦞 Ocean perch—raw ☞ 0 (Low)

🦞 Octopus—cooked, average value for cooking method ☞ 95 (High)

🦞 Octopus—dried, boiled ☞ 50 (Low)

🦞 Oysters—baked or broiled ☞ 50 (Low)

🦞 Oysters—battered, fried ☞ 95 (High)

🦞 Oysters—canned ☞ 50 (Low)

🦞 Oysters—floured or breaded, fried ☞ 95 (High)

🦞 Oysters—raw ☞ 50 (Low)

🦞 Oysters—smoked ☞ 50 (Low)

Oysters, cooked, average value for cooking method ☞ 95 (High)

Perch—baked or broiled ☞ 50 (Low)

Perch—battered, fried ☞ 95 (High)

Perch—breaded or battered, baked ☞ 95 (High)

Perch—cooked, average value for cooking method ☞ 95 (High)

Perch—floured or breaded, fried ☞ 95 (High)

Perch—steamed or poached ☞ 0 (Low)

Pike—baked or broiled ☞ 50 (Low)

Pompano—baked or broiled ☞ 50 (Low)

Pompano—floured or breaded, fried ☞ 95 (High)

Pompano—raw ☞ 0 (Low)

Porgy—baked or broiled ☞ 50 (Low)

Porgy—battered, fried ☞ 95 (High)

Porgy—breaded or battered, baked ☞ 95 (High)

Porgy—cooked, average value for cooking method ☞ 95 (High)

Porgy—floured or breaded, fried ☞ 95 (High)

Porgy—raw ☞ 0 (Low)

Porgy—steamed or poached ☞ 0 (Low)

Roe—cooked ☞ 50 (Low)

Roe—sturgeon ☞ 50 (Low)

Salmon—baked or broiled ☞ 50 (Low)

Salmon—battered, fried ☞ 95 (High)

Salmon—canned, oil or water ☞ 0 (Low)

Salmon—floured or breaded, fried ☞ 95 (High)

Salmon—smoked ☞ 0 (Low)

Salmon—steamed or poached ☞ 0 (Low)

Salmon, cooked, average value for cooking method ☞ 0 (Low)

Sardines—canned in oil ☞ 0 (Low)

Sardines—cooked ☞ 0 (Low)

Sardines—skinless, boneless, canned in water or oil ☞ 0 (Low)

Scallops—baked or broiled ☞ 50 (Low)

Scallops—battered, fried ☞ 95 (High)

Scallops—cooked, average value for cooking method ☞ 95 (High)

Scallops—floured or breaded, fried ☞ 95 (High)

Scallops—steamed or boiled ☞ 50 (Low)

Sea bass—baked or broiled ☞ 50 (Low)

Sea bass—floured or breaded, fried ☞ 95 (High)

Sea bass—steamed or poached ☞ 0 (Low)

Shark—steamed or poached ☞ 0 (Low)

Shrimp—baked or broiled ☞ 50 (Low)

Shrimp—canned, oil or water ☞ 50 (Low)

Shrimp—floured, fried ☞ 95 (High)

Shrimp—steamed or boiled ☞ 50 (Low)

Shrimp,—cooked, average value for cooking method ☞ 50 (Low)

Smelt—battered, fried ☞ 95 (High)

Smelt—floured or breaded, fried ☞ 95 (High)

🐌 Snails—cooked, average value for cooking method 🖙 50 (Low)

🦑 Squid—baked, broiled 🖙 50 (Low)

🦑 Squid—breaded, fried 🖙 95 (High)

🦑 Squid—canned in oil or water 🖙 50 (Low)

🦑 Squid—pickled 🖙 50 (Low)

🦑 Squid—steamed or boiled 🖙 50 (Low)

🐟 Swordfish—baked or broiled 🖙 50 (Low)

🐟 Swordfish—floured or breaded, fried 🖙 95 (High)

🐟 Swordfish—steamed or poached 🖙 0 (Low)

🐟 Swordfish, cooked, average value for cooking method 🖙 50 (Low)

🐟 Trout—baked or broiled 🖙 50 (Low)

🐟 Trout—battered, fried 🖙 95 (High)

🐟 Trout—breaded or battered, baked 🖙 95 (High)

🐟 Trout—floured or breaded, fried 🖙 95 (High)

🐟 Trout—smoked 🖙 0 (Low)

🐟 Trout—steamed or poached 🖙 0 (Low)

🐟 Tuna—canned, in oil or water 🖙 0 (Low)

🐟 Tuna—canned, in oil 🖙 0 (Low)

🐟 Tuna—canned, in water 🖙 0 (Low)

🐟 Tuna—fresh—baked or broiled 🖙 50 (Low)

🐟 Tuna—fresh—floured or breaded, fried 🖙 95 (High)

🐟 Tuna—fresh—steamed or poached 🖙 0 (Low)

🐟 Tuna—fresh, raw 🖙 0 (Low)

🦑 Whiting—baked or broiled ☛ 50 (Low)

🦑 Whiting—battered, fried ☛ 95 (High)

🦑 Whiting—floured or breaded, fried ☛ 95 (High)

19

FRUIT AND FRUIT PRODUCTS

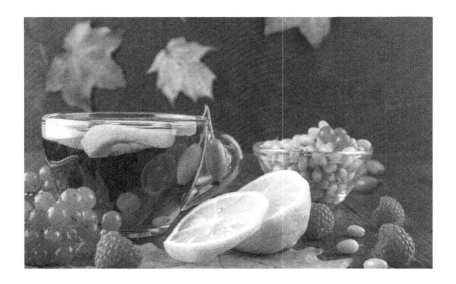

What is the serving size?

The typical serving sizes for low GI fruits and fruits juices are equivalent to:

- 1 medium piece of low GI or moderate GI fruit

- 1 cup of canned or sliced fruits
- 3/4 cup (6 oz) of fruit juice

For moderate GI fruits and fruits juices reduce the serving by 1/3

How Much a Day?

Up to 4 servings per day

Apple chips ☛ 38 (Low)

Apple—baked, Average value for added sweetener ☛ 38 (Low)

Apple—baked, unsweetened ☛ 38 (Low)

Apple—baked, with sugar ☛ 44 (Low)

Apple—candied ☛ 44 (Low)

Apple—chips ☛ 29 (Low)

Apple—cooked or canned, with light syrup ☛ 44 (Low)

Apple—dried ☛ 35 (Low)

Apple—dried, cooked, with sugar ☛ 29 (Low)

Apple—dried, uncooked ☛ 29 (Low)

Apple—fried ☛ 38 (Low)

Apple—peeled, common ☛ 38 (Low)

Apple—raw ☛ 38 (Low)

Apple, baked, no added sugar ☛ 38 (Low)

Apple, common ☛ 38 (Low)

Applesauce—stewed apples, Average value ☛ 38 (Low)

Applesauce—stewed apples, sweetened with low calorie sweetener ☛ 38 (Low)

Applesauce—stewed apples, unsweetened ☛ 38 (Low)

Applesauce—stewed apples, with sugar ☛ 38 (Low)

Apricot ☛ 31 (Low)

Apricot, dried, uncooked ☛ 31 (Low)

Apricots—dried ☛ 32 (Low)

Avocado ☛ 50 (Low)

Avocado—raw ☛ 50 (Low)

Banana—common, ripe ☛ 46-56 (Low)

Banana—dried ☛ 50 (Low)

Banana—raw ☛ 52 (Low)

Banana—red, ripe ☛ 52 (Low)

Banana—ripe, boiled ☛ 52 (Low)

Banana—ripe, fried ☛ 52 (Low)

Banana, chips ☛ 46-56 (Low)

Banana, common, firm ☛ 46-56 (Low)

Banana, raw ☛ 46-56 (Low)

Berries—raw, NFS ☛ 40 (Low)

Blackberry ☛ 25 (Low)

Blueberry ☛ 53 (Low)

Breadfruit ☛ 65 (Medium)

Cantaloupe ☛ 65 (Medium)

Cantaloupe—raw ☛ 65 (Medium)

Carambola—starfruit ☛ 45 (Low)

Cherries ☛ 22 (Low)

Cherries—frozen ☛ 22 (Low)

Cherries—sour, red, cooked, unsweetened ☛ 22 (Low)

Cherries—sweet—raw (Queen Anne, Bing) ☛ 22 (Low)

Cherries—sweet, cooked or canned, Average value ☛ 22 (Low)

Cherries—sweet, cooked or canned, drained solids ☛ 22 (Low)

Cherries—sweet, cooked or canned, in heavy syrup ☛ 22 (Low)

Cherries—sweet, cooked or canned, in light syrup ☛ 22 (Low)

Cherries—sweet, cooked or canned, juice pack ☛ 22 (Low)

Clementine ☛ 35 (Low)

Coconut ☛ 42 (Low)

Coconut—dried ☛ 45 (Low)

Cranberries—dried ☛ 45 (Low)

Currants ☛ 28 (Low)

Currants—dried ☛ 64 (Medium)

Currants—raw ☛ 64 (Medium)

Custard apple ☛ 54 (Low)

Date ☛ 103 (High)

Dates ☛ 44 (Low)

Durian ☛ 52 (Low)

Fig—dried, cooked, with sugar ☛ 61 (Medium)

Fig—dried, uncooked ☛ 61 (Medium)

Fig—raw ☛ 61 (Medium)

Figs—cooked or canned, in light syrup ☛ 61 (Medium)

Figs, dried ☛ 51 (Low)

Figs, dried ☛ 61 (Medium)

Figs, fresh ☛ 51 (Low)

Fruit cocktail (no citrus fruits)—raw ☛ 55 (Medium)

Fruit cocktail or mix (with citrus fruits)—raw ☛ 55 (Medium)

Fruit cocktail—cooked or canned, Average value ☛ 55 (Medium)

Fruit cocktail—cooked or canned, drained solids ☛ 55 (Medium)

Fruit cocktail—cooked or canned, in heavy syrup ☛ 55 (Medium)

Fruit cocktail—cooked or canned, in light syrup ☛ 55 (Medium)

Fruit cocktail—cooked or canned, juice pack ☛ 55 (Medium)

Fruit cocktail—cooked or canned, unsweetened, water pack ☛ 55 (Medium)

Fruit cocktail—frozen ☛ 55 (Medium)

Fruit juice bar—frozen, flavor other than orange ☛ 59 (Medium)

Fruit juice bar—frozen, orange flavor ☛ 59 (Medium)

Fruit juice bar—frozen, sweetened with low calorie sweetener, flavors other than orange ☛ 59 (Medium)

Fruit juice bar—with cream, frozen ☛ 42 (Low)

Fruit mixture—dried ☛ 38 (Low)

Fruit, dried—average value, excluding high glycemic fruits ☛ 38 (Low)

Goji berries—dried ☛ 30 (Low)

Grape, thompson ☞ 62 (Medium)

Grapefruit ☞ 25 (Low)

Grapefruit—canned or frozen, Average value ☞ 25 (Low)

Grapefruit—canned or frozen, in light syrup ☞ 25 (Low)

Grapefruit—canned or frozen, unsweetened, water pack ☞ 25 (Low)

Grapefruit—raw ☞ 25 (Low)

Grapes—American type, slip skin—raw ☞ 46 (Low)

Grapes—European type, adherent skin—raw ☞ 46 (Low)

Grapes—raw, Average value fo type ☞ 46 (Low)

Grapes, black ☞ 53 (Low)

Grapes, red ☞ 53 (Low)

Grapes, white ☞ 53 (Low)

Green Banana—cooked (in salt water) ☞ 38 (Low)

Green Banana—fried ☞ 30 (Low)

Green plantain—fried ☞ 39 (Low)

Green plantains—boiled ☞ 39 (Low)

Guacamole—with tomatoes ☞ 50 (Low)

Guacamole—with tomatoes and chili peppers ☞ 50 (Low)

Guacamole, average value ☞ 50 (Low)

Guava—immature/unriped ☞ 12 (Low)

Guava—mature/ripe ☞ 24 (Low)

Honeydew melon—raw ☞ 65 (Medium)

Honeydew—frozen ☞ 65 (Medium)

Ice fruit ☞ 59 (Medium)

Jackfruit—dried ☞ 60 (Medium)

Kiwi fruit—raw ☞ 53 (Low)

Kiwifruit—gold ☞ 43 (Low)

Kiwifruit—green ☞ 39 (Low)

Kumquat ☞ 0.0 (Low)

Kumquat, peeled ☞ 0.0 (Low)

Lemon, juice ☞ 28 (Low)

Lime, juice ☞ 20 (Low)

Lychee ☞ 50 (Low)

Mandarin—orange ☞ 47 (Low)

Mango ☞ 51 (Low)

Mango—dried ☞ 55 (Low)

Mangosteen ☞ 53 (Low)

Mangosteen—dried ☞ 62 (Medium)

Melon ☞ 62 (Medium)

Nectarine ☞ 46 (Low)

Nectarine—raw ☞ 42 (Low)

Orange—navel ☞ 42 (Low)

Orange—raw ☞ 42 (Low)

Orange, mandarin—canned or frozen, drained ☞ 42 (Low)

Orange, mandarin—canned or frozen, in light syrup ☞ 42 (Low)

Papaya ☞ 60 (Medium)

🍎 Papaya—cooked or canned 🐖 59 (Medium)

🍎 Papaya—dried 🐖 60 (Medium)

🍎 Papaya—green, cooked 🐖 59 (Medium)

🍎 Papaya—raw 🐖 59 (Medium)

🍎 Passion fruit 🐖 54 (Low)

🍎 Passionfruit 🐖 30 (Low)

🍎 Peach—canned or cooked, in heavy syrup 🐖 58 (Medium)

🍎 Peach—canned or cooked, in light or medium syrup 🐖 52 (Low)

🍎 Peach—common 🐖 42 (Low)

🍎 Peach—cooked or canned 🐖 42 (Low)

🍎 Peach—cooked or canned, Average value 🐖 58 (Medium)

🍎 Peach—cooked or canned, juice pack 🐖 38 (Low)

🍎 Peach—frozen, Average value fo added sweetener 🐖 58 (Medium)

🍎 Peach—frozen, unsweetened 🐖 42 (Low)

🍎 Peach—raw 🐖 42 (Low)

🍎 Peach—white 🐖 42 (Low)

🍎 Peach—yellow 🐖 42 (Low)

🍎 Peach, frozen, with sugar 🐖 58 (Medium)

🍎 Peaches 🐖 38 (Low)

🍎 Pear—cooked or canned 🐖 38 (Low)

🍎 Pear—cooked or canned, Average value 🐖 44 (Low)

🍎 Pear—cooked or canned, in heavy syrup 🐖 44 (Low)

🍎 Pear—cooked or canned, in light syrup 🐖 25 (Low)

- Pear—cooked or canned, juice pack ☛ 44 (Low)

- Pear—dried ☛ 48 (Low)

- Pear—Japanese—raw ☛ 38 (Low)

- Pear—nashi ☛ 30 (Low)

- Pear—prickly ☛ 40 (Low)

- Pear—raw ☛ 38 (Low)

- Pear—ripe, peeled ☛ 30 (Low)

- Pear—unripe peeled ☛ 28 (Low)

- Persimmon ☛ 61 (Medium)

- Pineapple ☛ 66 (Medium)

- PineApple—cooked or canned, Average value ☛ 59 (Medium)

- PineApple—cooked or canned, drained solids ☛ 59 (Medium)

- PineApple—cooked or canned, in heavy syrup ☛ 59 (Medium)

- PineApple—cooked or canned, in light syrup ☛ 59 (Medium)

- PineApple—cooked or canned, juice pack ☛ 59 (Medium)

- PineApple—cooked or canned, unsweetened ☛ 59 (Medium)

- Pineapple—dried ☛ 62 (Medium)

- Pineapple—raw ☛ 59 (Medium)

- Plaintain—peeled ☛ 37 (Low)

- Plantain—boiled, Average value for green or ripe ☛ 39 (Low)

- Plantain—fried, Average value for green or ripe ☛ 39 (Low)

- Plum ☛ 40 (Low)

- Plum—cooked or canned, in heavy syrup ☛ 39 (Low)

Plum—cooked or canned, in light syrup ☞ 39 (Low)

Plum—raw ☞ 39 (Low)

Pomegranate ☞ 53 (Low)

Prune—dried, cooked, unsweetened ☞ 29 (Low)

Prune—dried, cooked, without sugar ☞ 29 (Low)

Prune—dried, uncooked ☞ 29 (Low)

Prune, dried, cooked, Average value ☞ 29 (Low)

Prunes ☞ 40 (Low)

Raisins ☞ 64 (Medium)

Raisins ☞ 64 (Medium)

Raisins—cooked ☞ 64 (Medium)

Rambutan ☞ 60 (Medium)

Raspberry ☞ 32 (Low)

Rhubarb ☞ 16 (Low)

Sorbet fruit—citrus flavor ☞ 59 (Medium)

Sorbet fruit—noncitrus flavor ☞ 59 (Medium)

Starfruit ☞ 45 (Low)

Strawberries—cooked or canned, Average value ☞ 55 (Low)

Strawberries—cooked or canned, in syrup ☞ 55 (Low)

Strawberries—frozen, Average value ☞ 55 (Low)

Strawberries—frozen, unsweetened ☞ 40 (Low)

Strawberries—frozen, with sugar ☞ 55 (Low)

Strawberries—raw ☞ 40 (Low)

- Strawberries—raw, with sugar ☛ 55 (Low)

- Strawberry ☛ 41 (Low)

- Sultanas ☛ 56 (Medium)

- Tamarind ☛ 22 (Low)

- Tangelo—raw ☛ 42 (Low)

- Tangerine—raw ☛ 42 (Low)

- Watermelon ☛ 72 (High)

20

GRAINS & BREAKFAST CEREALS

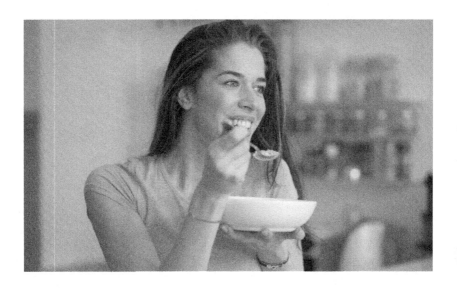

What is the serving size?

The typical serving sizes for low GI Breakfast Cereals are equivalent to:

- ⅓ cup breakfast cereal or muesli

- ½ cup of cooked cereal, pasta, or other cooked grain
- ⅓ cup of cooked rice, and other small grains
- ¾ cup of cold cereal

For moderate GI Grains & Breakfast Cereals reduce the serving by 1/3

How Much a Day?

Up to 8 servings per day provided you respect your calorie deficit in your overall daily intake.

Barleypearl ☛ 25 (Low)

Bran, oat, whole ☛ 55 (Low)

Bran, rice, whole ☛ 65 (Medium)

Bran, wheat, minimally processed ☛ 55 (Low)

Bran, wheat, whole ☛ 55 (Low)

Buckwheat kernals ☛ 35 (Low)

Buckwheat, groats ☛ 35 (Low)

Bulgur ☛ 48 (Low)

Corn cob ☛ 52 (Low)

Corn, popcorn ☛ 65 (Medium)

Corn, tortilla ☛ 46 (Low)

Couscous, mainly from rice and corn ☛ 65 (Medium)

Flour—Almond ☛ 0-1 (Low)

Flour—Amaranth ☛ 105 (High)

Flour—Barley ☛ 25 (Low)

🐦 Flour—Buckwheat 🐀 35 (Low)

🐦 Flour—Chestnut 🐀 65 (Medium)

🐦 Flour—Coconut 🐀 51 (Low)

🐦 Flour—Corn 🐀 87 (High)

🐦 Flour—Corn, yellow 🐀 87 (High)

🐦 Flour—Einkorn 🐀 48 (Low)

🐦 Flour—Emmer 🐀 42 (Low)

🐦 Flour—Kamut, (Khorasan) 🐀 40 (Low)

🐦 Flour—Maize 🐀 94 (High)

🐦 Flour—Maize, starch 🐀 94 (High)

🐦 Flour—Millet 🐀 53 (Low)

🐦 Flour—Potato, starch 🐀 85 (High)

🐦 Flour—Quinoa 🐀 53 (Low)

🐦 Flour—Rye 🐀 65 (Medium)

🐦 Flour—Rye 🐀 65 (Medium)

🐦 Flour—Sorgham 🐀 64 (Medium)

🐦 Flour—Tapioca, starch 🐀 65 (Medium)

🐦 Flour—Teff 🐀 36 (Low)

🐦 Flour—White Spelt 🐀 63 (Medium)

🐦 Flour—White Wheat 🐀 85 (High)

🐦 Flour—Whole-Wheat 🐀 69 (Medium)

🐦 Flour—Yam 🐀 51 (Low)

🐦 Millet, grains 🐀 53 (Low)

Millet, hulled ☞ 53 (Low)

Oat, flakes ☞ 55 (Low)

Oats, whole ☞ 55 (Low)

Quinoa grain ☞ 53 (Low)

Quinoa, black ☞ 53 (Low)

Quinoa, red ☞ 53 (Low)

Quinoa, white ☞ 53 (Low)

Rice, Basmati ☞ 52-59 (Low)

Rice, brown ☞ 55 (Low)

Rice, white ☞ 73 (High)

Spelt, green ☞ 93 (High)

100% Bran ☞ 42 (Low)

All-Bran ☞ 42 (Low)

All-Bran with Extra Fiber ☞ 42 (Low)

Apple Cinnamon Cheerios ☞ 74 (High)

Apple Cinnamon Oh's Cereal ☞ 74 (High)

Apple Cinnamon Rice Krispies ☞ 82 (High)

Barley—cooked, with fat ☞ 25 (Low)

Barley—cooked, without fat ☞ 25 (Low)

Berry Berry Kix ☞ 113 (High)

Bran Chex ☞ 58 (Low)

Bran Flakes ☞ 74 (High)

Breakfast bar—cake-like ☞ 57 (Medium)

Breakfast bar—cereal crust with fruit ☛ 72 (High)

Breakfast bar—cereal crust with fruit, low fat ☛ 72 (High)

Breakfast bar—Common ☛ 57 (Medium)

Breakfast bar—date, yogurt coating ☛ 53.5 (Low)

Breakfast bar—diet ☛ 39.3 (Low)

Buckwheat groats—cooked, with fat ☛ 45 (Low)

Buckwheat groats—cooked, without fat ☛ 45 (Low)

Bulgur—canned, average value ☛ 48 (Low)

Bulgur—canned, with fat ☛ 48 (Low)

Bulgur—canned, without fat ☛ 48 (Low)

Bulgur—cooked or canned, average value ☛ 48 (Low)

Bulgur—cooked or canned, with fat ☛ 48 (Low)

Bulgur—cooked or canned, without fat ☛ 48 (Low)

Cereal—average value ☛ 74.6 (High)

Cereal—ready-to-eat, average value ☛ 74.6 (High)

Cheerios ☛ 74 (High)

Chex cereal—average value ☛ 58 (Medium)

Cocoa Krispies ☛ 77 (High)

Cocoa Pebbles ☛ 77 (High)

Cocoa Puffs ☛ 80 (High)

Corn flakes (average value) ☛ 81 (High)

Corn—canned, yellow, low-sodium, with fat ☛ 46 (Low)

Corn—canned, yellow, low-sodium, without fat ☛ 46 (Low)

Corn—cooked, average (fresh, frozen, canned) 🐾 53.5 (Low)

Corn—cooked, average (fresh, frozen, canned), cream style 🐾 53.5 (Low)

Corn—cooked, average (fresh, frozen, canned), with cream sauce 🐾 46.2 (Low)

Corn—cooked, average (fresh, frozen, canned), with fat 🐾 53.5 (Low)

Corn—cooked, average (fresh, frozen, canned), without fat 🐾 53.5 (Low)

Corn—from canned cooked, not specified if fat is added 🐾 46 (Low)

Corn—from canned, cooked, white, average 🐾 46 (Low)

Corn—from canned, cooked, white, with fat 🐾 46 (Low)

Corn—from canned, cooked, white, without fat 🐾 46 (Low)

Corn—from canned, cooked, with fat 🐾 46 (Low)

Corn—from canned, cooked, without fat 🐾 46 (Low)

Corn—from canned, cooked, yellow 🐾 46 (Low)

Corn—from canned, cooked, yellow and white, without fat 🐾 46 (Low)

Corn—from canned, cooked, yellow, with fat 🐾 46 (Low)

Corn—from canned, cooked, yellow, without fat 🐾 46 (Low)

Corn—from canned, white, cream style 🐾 46 (Low)

Corn—from canned, yellow, cream style 🐾 46 (Low)

Corn—from canned, yellow, with fat, cream style 🐾 46 (Low)

Corn—from fresh cooked, NS as to color, fat not added in cooking 🐾 53.5 (Low)

Corn—from fresh cooked, with fat ☞ 53.5 (Low)

Corn—from fresh, cooked (average) ☞ 53.5 (Low)

Corn—from fresh, cooked, cream sauce ☞ 46.2 (Low)

Corn—from fresh, cooked, white, average ☞ 53.5 (Low)

Corn—from fresh, cooked, white, with fat ☞ 53.5 (Low)

Corn—from fresh, cooked, white, without fat ☞ 53.5 (Low)

Corn—from fresh, cooked, yellow ☞ 53.5 (Low)

Corn—from fresh, cooked, yellow and white ☞ 53.5 (Low)

Corn—from fresh, cooked, yellow and white, with fat ☞ 53.5 (Low)

Corn—from fresh, cooked, yellow and white, without fat ☞ 53.5 (Low)

Corn—from fresh, cooked, yellow, with fat ☞ 53.5 (Low)

Corn—from fresh, cooked, yellow, without fat ☞ 53.5 (Low)

Corn—from frozen, cooked (average) ☞ 47 (Low)

Corn—from frozen, cooked, cream sauce ☞ 46.2 (Low)

Corn—from frozen, cooked, white, average ☞ 53.5 (Low)

Corn—from frozen, cooked, white, with fat ☞ 47 (Low)

Corn—from frozen, cooked, white, without fat ☞ 47 (Low)

Corn—from frozen, cooked, with fat ☞ 47 (Low)

Corn—from frozen, cooked, without fat ☞ 47 (Low)

Corn—from frozen, cooked, yellow ☞ 47 (Low)

Corn—from frozen, cooked, yellow and white ☞ 47 (Low)

Corn—from frozen, cooked, yellow and white, without fat ☞ 47 (Low)

Corn—from frozen, cooked, yellow, with fat ☛ 47 (Low)

Corn—from frozen, cooked, yellow, without fat ☛ 47 (Low)

Corn—raw ☛ 53.5 (Low)

Corn—white, cooked, average (fresh, frozen, canned) ☛ 53.5 (Low)

Corn—yellow and white, cooked, with fat ☛ 53.5 (Low)

Corn—yellow and white, cooked, without fat ☛ 53.5 (Low)

Corn—yellow, cooked, average value ☛ 53.5 (Low)

Corn—yellow, cooked, average value, with fat ☛ 53.5 (Low)

Corn—yellow, cooked, average value, without fat ☛ 53.5 (Low)

Crispix ☛ 87 (High)

Crispy Brown Rice ☛ 82 (High)

Crispy Rice ☛ 82 (High)

Crispy Wheats'n-Raisins ☛ 61 (Medium)

Flavored rice—brown and wild ☛ 54 (Low)

Flavored rice—mixture ☛ 54.7 (Low)

Flavored rice—white and wild ☛ 54 (Low)

Frosted Cheerios ☛ 74 (High)

Kellogg's—All-Bran Bran Buds ☛ 58 (Medium)

Kellogg's—Almond Crunch with raisins Healthy Choice ☛ 68 (Medium)

Kellogg's—Apple Cinnamon Squares ☛ 58 (Medium)

Kellogg's—Complete Wheat Bran ☛ 74 (High)

Kellogg's—Corn flakes ☛ 81 (High)

Kellogg's—Frosted Flakes ☛ 55 (Low)

Kellogg's—Frosted Mini-Wheats ☞ 58 (Medium)

Kellogg's—Frosted Wheat Bites ☞ 72 (High)

Kellogg's—Honey Crunch Corn Flakes ☞ 72 (High)

Kellogg's—Multi-Grain Flakes Healthy Choice ☞ 68 (Medium)

Kellogg's—Multi-Grain Squares Healthy Choice ☞ 70 (High)

Kellogg's—Raisin Bran ☞ 61 (Medium)

Kellogg's—Raisin Squares Mini Wheats ☞ 65 (Medium)

Kellogg's—Rice Krispies Treats Cereal ☞ 82 (High)

Kellogg's—Strawberry Squares Mini-Wheats ☞ 72 (High)

Oat bran—cooked, milk, without fat ☞ 44.2 (Low)

Oat bran—cooked, with fat ☞ 55 (Low)

Oat bran—cooked, without fat ☞ 55 (Low)

Oat Bran—plain Common Sense ☞ 77 (High)

Oat Bran—raisins, Common Sense ☞ 77 (High)

Oat cereal—common ☞ 74 (High)

Oat flakes—fortified ☞ 67 (Medium)

Oat Flakes—Health Valley ☞ 67 (Medium)

Oat Flakes—Post ☞ 67 (Medium)

Oatmeal—cooked, fortified, instant or quick, with fat ☞ 58 (Medium)

Oatmeal—cooked, fortified, instant or quick, without fat ☞ 58 (Medium)

Oatmeal—cooked, instant, average ☞ 58 (Medium)

Oatmeal—cooked, instant, with fat ☞ 58 (Medium)

Oatmeal—cooked, instant, without fat ☛ 58 (Medium)

Oatmeal—cooked, multigrain, without fat ☛ 58 (Medium)

Oatmeal—cooked, oat bran, instant, without fat ☛ 58 (Medium)

Oatmeal—cooked, quick or instant, average value ☛ 58 (Medium)

Oatmeal—cooked, quick or instant, with fat ☛ 58 (Medium)

Oatmeal—cooked, quick or instant, without fat ☛ 58 (Medium)

Oatmeal—cooked, regular, average value ☛ 58 (Medium)

Oatmeal—cooked, regular, with fat ☛ 58 (Medium)

Oatmeal—cooked, regular, without fat ☛ 58 (Medium)

Oatmeal—cooked, with flavors ☛ 58 (Medium)

Oatmeal—cooked, with fruit ☛ 58 (Medium)

Oatmeal—Crisp with Almonds ☛ 77 (High)

Rice—brown and wild, cooked, fat added in cooking ☛ 54 (Low)

Rice—brown and wild, cooked, fat not added in cooking ☛ 54 (Low)

Rice—brown and wild, cooked, NS as to fat added in cooking ☛ 54 (Low)

Rice—brown, cooked, instant, fat added in cooking ☛ 64 (Medium)

Rice—brown, cooked, instant, fat not added in cooking ☛ 64 (Medium)

Rice—brown, cooked, instant, NS as to fat added in cooking ☛ 55 (Low)

Rice—brown, cooked, regular, fat added in cooking ☛ 55 (Low)

Rice—brown, cooked, regular, fat not added in cooking ☛ 55 (Low)

Rice—brown, cooked, regular, NS as to fat added in cooking ☛ 55 (Low)

Rice—cooked, NFS ☛ 64 (Medium)

Rice—cooked, NS as to type, fat added in cooking ☛ 64 (Medium)

Rice—cream of, cooked, fat not added in cooking ☛ 64 (Medium)

Rice—puffed ☛ 87 (High)

Rice—white and wild, cooked, fat added in cooking ☛ 54 (Low)

Rice—white and wild, cooked, fat not added in cooking ☛ 54 (Low)

Rice—white and wild, cooked, NS as to fat added in cooking ☛ 54 (Low)

Rice—white, cooked with (fat) oil, Puerto Rican style (Arroz blanco) ☛ 64 (Medium)

Rice—white, cooked, converted, fat added in cooking ☛ 47 (Low)

Rice—white, cooked, converted, fat not added in cooking ☛ 47 (Low)

Rice—white, cooked, converted, NS as to fat added in cooking ☛ 47 (Low)

Rice—white, cooked, glutinous ☛ 98 (High)

Rice—white, cooked, instant, fat added in cooking ☛ 69 (Medium)

Rice—white, cooked, instant, fat not added in cooking ☛ 69 (Medium)

Rice—white, cooked, instant, NS as to fat added in cooking ☛ 69 (Medium)

Rice—white, cooked, regular, fat added in cooking ☞ 64 (Medium)

Rice—white, cooked, regular, fat not added in cooking ☞ 64 (Medium)

Rice—white, cooked, regular, NS as to fat added in cooking ☞ 64 (Medium)

Rice—wild, 100%, cooked, fat not added in cooking ☞ 57 (Medium)

21

LEGUMES AND NUTS

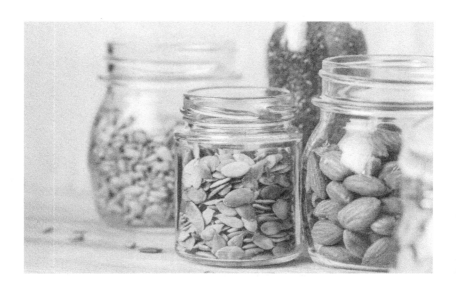

What is the serving size?

The typical serving sizes for low GI legumes and nuts are equivalent to:

- ⅓ cup of nuts (5 large or 10 small nuts)
- ½ cup of cooked or canned beans, lentils, and chickpeas
- 2 tablespoons of nut butter
- 2 tablespoons of nut spread

For moderate GI Legumes and Nuts reduce the serving by 1/3

Baked beans fresh—boiled ☞ 40 (Low)

Baked beans—low sodium ☞ 48 (Low)

Baked beans—NFS ☞ 48 (Low)

Baked beans—with pork and sweet sauce ☞ 48 (Low)

Baked beans—with tomato sauce ☞ 48 (Low)

Bayo Beans—dry, cooked ☞ 20 (Low)

Bayo Beans—dry, cooked, with fat ☞ 20 (Low)

Bayo Beans—dry, cooked, without fat ☞ 20 (Low)

Beans green string—with onions, cooked, with fat ☞ 32 (Low)

Beans lima—immature, canned ☞ 32 (Low)

Beans lima—immature, cooked ☞ 32 (Low)

Beans lima—immature, cooked, from canned ☞ 32 (Low)

Beans lima—immature, cooked, from canned, with fat ☞ 32 (Low)

Beans lima—immature, cooked, from canned, without fat ☞ 32 (Low)

Beans lima—immature, cooked, from fresh, with fat ☞ 32 (Low)

Beans lima—immature, cooked, from fresh, without fat ☞ 32 (Low)

Beans lima—immature, cooked, from frozen ☞ 32 (Low)

Beans lima—immature, cooked, from frozen, with fat ☞ 32 (Low)

Beans lima—immature, cooked, from frozen, without fat ☞ 32 (Low)

Beans lima—immature, cooked, with fat ☞ 32 (Low)

Beans lima—immature, cooked, without fat ☞ 32 (Low)

Beans lima—immature, from frozen, creamed or with cheese sauce ☞ 31 (Low)

Beans string—cooked, from canned, with fat ☞ 32 (Low)

Beans string—cooked, from fresh, with fat ☞ 32 (Low)

Beans string—cooked, from frozen, with fat ☞ 32 (Low)

Beans string—cooked, with fat ☞ 32 (Low)

Beans string—green, canned, with fat ☞ 32 (Low)

Beans string—green, cooked, from canned, with fat ☞ 32 (Low)

Beans string—green, cooked, from fresh, with fat ☞ 32 (Low)

Beans string—green, cooked, from frozen, with fat ☞ 32 (Low)

Beans string—green, cooked, with fat ☞ 32 (Low)

Beans string—green, raw ☞ 32 (Low)

Beans string—yellow, cooked, from canned, with fat ☞ 32 (Low)

Beans string—yellow, cooked, from fresh, with fat ☞ 32 (Low)

Beans string—yellow, cooked, from frozen, with fat ☞ 32 (Low)

Beans string—yellow, cooked, with fat ☞ 32 (Low)

Beans—dry, cooked with ground beef ☞ 48 (Low)

Beans—dry, cooked with pork ☛ 48 (Low)

Beans—dry, cooked, average value for added fat ☛ 29 (Low)

Beans—dry, cooked, with fat ☛ 29 (Low)

Beans—dry, cooked, with fat ☛ 29 (Low)

Black beans—canned ☛ 20 (Low)

Black beans, fresh—boiled ☛ 20 (Low)

Boston baked beans ☛ 48 (Low)

Butter beans—canned ☛ 31 (Low)

Butter beans—fresh ☛ 31 (Low)

Cannellini beans fresh—boiled ☛ 32 (Low)

Cannellini beans—canned ☛ 32 (Low)

Chana dal fresh—boiled ☛ 8 (Low)

Chickpeas fresh—boiled ☛ 28 (Low)

Chickpeas— dry, cooked ☛ 28 (Low)

Chickpeas— dry, cooked, with fat ☛ 28 (Low)

Chickpeas— dry, cooked, without fat ☛ 28 (Low)

Chickpeas— stewed with pig's feet, Puerto Rican style (Garbanzos guisados con patitos de cerdo) ☛ 28 (Low)

Chickpeas—canned ☛ 28 (Low)

Chili Beans ☛ 48 (Low)

Cowpeas— dry, cooked ☛ 42 (Low)

Cowpeas— dry, cooked with pork ☛ 42 (Low)

Cowpeas— dry, cooked, with fat ☛ 42 (Low)

🌿 Cowpeas— dry, cooked, without fat ☞ 42 (Low)

🌿 Fava (Broad) beans fresh—boiled ☞ 79 (High)

🌿 Fava (broad) beans—canned ☞ 79 (High)

🌿 Garbanzo beans—canned ☞ 28 (Low)

🌿 Green or yellow split peas—dry, cooked ☞ 32 (Low)

🌿 Green or yellow split peas—dry, cooked, without fat ☞ 32 (Low)

🌿 Lentils—canned ☞ 32 (Low)

🌿 Lentils—dry, cooked ☞ 28 (Low)

🌿 Lentils—dry, cooked, with fat ☞ 28 (Low)

🌿 Lentils—dry, cooked, without fat ☞ 28 (Low)

🌿 Lentils, green—canned ☞ 32 (Low)

🌿 Lentils, green, fresh—boiled ☞ 32 (Low)

🌿 Lentils, red—canned ☞ 32 (Low)

🌿 Lentils, red, fresh—boiled ☞ 32 (Low)

🌿 Lima beans—canned ☞ 46 (Low)

🌿 Lima Beans—dry, cooked ☞ 31 (Low)

🌿 Lima Beans—dry, cooked, with fat ☞ 31 (Low)

🌿 Lima Beans—dry, cooked, without fat ☞ 31 (Low)

🌿 Lima Beans—Stewed, dry ☞ 31 (Low)

🌿 Lima Beans—Stewed, dry -Habichuelas coloradas guisadas ☞ 28 (Low)

🌿 Lima beans, fresh—boiled ☞ 46 (Low)

🌿 Motley beans fresh—boiled ☞ 35 (Low)

🌿 Motley beans—canned ☞ 35 (Low)

🌿 Mung beans—canned ☛ 31 (Low)

🌿 Mung Beans—with fat ☛ 37 (Low)

🌿 Mung Beans—without fat ☛ 37 (Low)

🌿 Mung beans, fresh—boiled ☛ 31 (Low)

🌿 Navy beans, fresh—boiled ☛ 39 (Low)

🌿 Peas, Cowpeas—cooked, from fresh ☛ 42 (Low)

🌿 Pinto beans dry ☛ 39 (Low)

🌿 Pinto beans—canned ☛ 39 (Low)

🌿 Pinto Beans—dry, cooked ☛ 39 (Low)

🌿 Pinto Beans—dry, cooked, with fat ☛ 39 (Low)

🌿 Pinto Beans—dry, cooked, without fat ☛ 39 (Low)

🌿 Pork and beans ☛ 48 (Low)

🌿 Red kidney beans fresh—boiled ☛ 24 (Low)

🌿 Red kidney Beans—dry, cooked ☛ 28 (Low)

🌿 Red kidney Beans—dry, cooked, with fat ☛ 28 (Low)

🌿 Red kidney Beans—dry, cooked, without fat ☛ 28 (Low)

🌿 Refried beans ☛ 42 (Low)

🌿 Soya beans, fresh—boiled ☛ 14 (Low)

🌿 Soybean curd ☛ 16 (Low)

🌿 Soybean curd—breaded, fried ☛ 16 (Low)

🌿 Soybean curd—deep fried ☛ 16 (Low)

🌿 Soybean meal ☛ 16 (Low)

🌿 SoyBeans—cooked, with fat ☛ 16 (Low)

Soyburger—meatless, without bun ☞ 16 (Low)

Split peas, fresh—boiled ☞ 32 (Low)

White Beans—dry, cooked ☞ 13 (Low)

White Beans—dry, cooked, with fat ☞ 13 (Low)

White Beans—dry, cooked, without fat ☞ 13 (Low)

22

MIXED MEALS AND CONVENIENCE FOODS

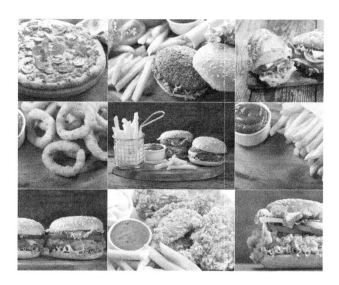

Featuring 200+ more new listings in the category "mixed meals and convenience foods", this essential 2021 reference table provides the GI counts you need to know for generic and brand-name foods. Data were compiled from the most authoritative sources, and some GI values were calculated as the mean of up to five studies.

Bacon—average value concerning meat, cooked ☞ 50 (Low)

Bacon—or side pork, fresh, cooked ☞ 50 (Low)

Bacon—Pork formed, lean meat added, cooked ☞ 50 (Low)

Bacon—Pork NS as to fresh, smoked or cured, cooked ☞ 50 (Low)

Bacon—Pork smoked or cured, cooked ☞ 50 (Low)

Bacon—Pork smoked or cured, cooked, lean only eaten ☞ 50 (Low)

Bacon—Pork smoked or cured, lower sodium ☞ 50 (Low)

Beef and noodles—with tomato sauce ☞ 40 (Low)

Beef and vegetables—carrots, broccoli, dark-green leafy, soy-based sauce ☞ 49 (Low)

Beef noodle soup ☞ 42 (Low)

Beef noodle soup—home recipe ☞ 42 (Low)

Beef noodle soup—Sopa de carne y fideos ☞ 42 (Low)

Beef pot pie ☞ 45 (Low)

Beef pot pie ☞ 45 (Low)

Beef rice soup ☞ 64 (Medium)

Beef sausage— Average Value ☞ 28 (Low)

Beef sausage— brown and serve, links, cooked ☞ 28 (Low)

Beef sausage— fresh, bulk, patty or link, cooked ☞ 28 (Low)

Beef sausage— smoked ☞ 28 (Low)

Beef sausage— smoked, stick ☞ 28 (Low)

Beef stew—with potatoes, tomato sauce ☞ 70 (Medium)

Beef stroganoff soup—chunky style ☞ 42 (Low)

Beef stroganoff—with noodles ☞ 46 (Low)

Beef stroganoff—with noodles ☞ 46 (Low)

Beef vegetable soup—Sopa caldo de Res ☞ 38 (Low)

Beef vegetable soup—with noodles, stew type, chunky style ☞ 40 (Low)

Beef vegetable soup—with potato, stew type ☞ 44 (Low)

Beef vegetable soup—with rice, stew type, chunky style ☞ 51 (Low)

Beef vegetables stew—potatoes, carrots, broccoli, dark-green leafy, tomato sauce ☞ 63 (Medium)

Beef vegetables stew—potatoes, carrots, broccoli, dark-green leafy ☞ 64 (Medium)

Beef—sloppy joe without bun ☞ 42 (Low)

Beef—with barbecue sauce ☞ 38 (Low)

Beef—with gravy ☞ 71 (High)

Beef—with tomato sauce ☞ 37 (Low)

Beef, bacon— cooked ☞ 50 (Low)

Beef, bacon— formed, lean meat added, cooked ☞ 50 (Low)

Beef, rice, and vegetables soup —not carrots, not broccoli ☞ 49 (Low)

Beef, rice, and vegetables soup—with carrots, broccoli ☞ 47 (Low)

Black bean soup ☞ 64 (Medium)

Blood sausage ☞ 28 (Low)

Bologna ring—smoked ☞ 28 (Low)

📖 Bologna— Average Value ☞ 28 (Low)

📖 Bologna— beef ☞ 28 (Low)

📖 Bologna— beef and pork, lowfat ☞ 28 (Low)

📖 Bologna— beef, lower sodium ☞ 28 (Low)

📖 Bologna— beef, lowfat ☞ 28 (Low)

📖 Bologna— chicken, beef, and pork ☞ 28 (Low)

📖 Bologna— Lebanon ☞ 28 (Low)

📖 Bologna— pork ☞ 28 (Low)

📖 Bologna— pork and beef ☞ 28 (Low)

📖 Bologna— turkey ☞ 28 (Low)

📖 Bratwurst, cooked ☞ 28 (Low)

📖 Broccoli cheese soup—prepared with milk ☞ 27 (Low)

📖 Broccoli soup ☞ 27 (Low)

📖 Burrito—beef, with beans, sour cream and cheese ☞ 33 (Low)

📖 Burrito—sausage, cheese, eggs and vegetables ☞ 31 (Low)

📖 Burrito—with beef and beans ☞ 34 (Low)

📖 Burrito—with beef and cheese, whitout beans ☞ 30 (Low)

📖 Burrito—with beef, with beans, and cheese ☞ 34 (Low)

📖 Burrito—with cheese, beans, without meat or poultry ☞ 34 (Low)

📖 Canadian bacon, cooked ☞ 50 (Low)

📖 Carrot soup—prepared with milk ☞ 37 (Low)

📖 Cauliflower soup—prepared with milk ☞ 27 (Low)

📖 Celery soup—made with milk or water, average value ☞ 27 (Low)

📖 Celery soup—prepared with milk ☛ 27 (Low)

📖 Celery soup—prepared with water ☛ 27 (Low)

📖 Cheddar cheese soup ☛ 27 (Low)

📖 Chicken and Beef sausage— smoked ☛ 28 (Low)

📖 Chicken and mushroom soup—prepared with milk ☛ 27 (Low)

📖 Chicken and noodles—no sauce ☛ 40 (Low)

📖 Chicken and noodles—with cream or white sauce ☛ 46 (Low)

📖 Chicken fillet sandwich—broiled, cheese, lettuce, tomato, spread, and bun ☛ 59 (Medium)

📖 Chicken fillet sandwich—broiled, lettuce, tomato, spread and whole-wheat roll ☛ 69 (Medium)

📖 Chicken garden salad—tomato, carrots, other vegetables, no potato, no dressing ☛ 32 (Low)

📖 Chicken gumbo soup ☛ 38 (Low)

📖 Chicken or turkey—cacciatore ☛ 61 (Medium)

📖 Chicken or turkey—cordon bleu ☛ 82 (High)

📖 Chicken parmigiana ☛ 79 (High)

📖 Chicken patty sandwich ☛ 67 (Medium)

📖 Chicken pot pie ☛ 85 (High)

📖 Chicken salad ☛ 41 (Low)

📖 Chicken teriyaki ☛ 57 (Medium)

📖 Chicken with barbecue sauce ☛ 38 (Low)

📖 Chicken with dumplings ☛ 91 (High)

📖 Chicken with vegetables—carrots, broccoli, dark-green leafy without sauce ☛ 43 (Low)

📖 Chicken with vegetables—carrots, broccoli, dark-green leafy, with soy-based sauce ☞ 55 (Low)

📖 Chiles rellenos ☞ 35 (Low)

📖 Chili con carne—beans ☞ 34 (Low)

📖 Chili con carne—beans and cheese ☞ 34 (Low)

📖 Chili con carne—beans and rice ☞ 55 (Low)

📖 Chili con carne—beans, macaroni ☞ 41 (Low)

📖 Chili con carne—beans, made with chicken ☞ 34 (Low)

📖 Chili con carne—beans, made with turkey ☞ 34 (Low)

📖 Chili con carne—beans, made with venison/deer ☞ 34 (Low)

📖 Chili con carne—beans, prepared with pork ☞ 34 (Low)

📖 Chili con carne—without beans ☞ 37 (Low)

📖 Chorizos ☞ 28 (Low)

📖 Cold cut—Average Value ☞ 28 (Low)

📖 Deer bologna ☞ 28 (Low)

📖 Fajita with chicken and vegetables ☞ 31 (Low)

📖 Frankfurter, Wiener, or Hot Dog—beef ☞ 28 (Low)

📖 Frankfurter, Wiener, or Hot Dog—beef and pork ☞ 28 (Low)

📖 Frankfurter, Wiener, or Hot Dog—beef and pork, lowfat ☞ 28 (Low)

📖 Frankfurter, Wiener, or Hot Dog—beef, lowfat ☞ 28 (Low)

📖 Frankfurter, Wiener, or Hot Dog—chicken ☞ 28 (Low)

📖 Frankfurter, Wiener, or Hot Dog—low salt ☞ 28 (Low)

📖 Frankfurter, Wiener, or Hot Dog—meat & poultry, lowfat ☞

28 (Low)

📖 Frankfurter, Wiener, or Hot Dog—meat and poultry ☞ 28 (Low)

📖 Frankfurter, Wiener, or Hot Dog—meat and poultry, fat free ☞ 28 (Low)

📖 Frankfurter, Wiener, or Hot Dog—turkey ☞ 28 (Low)

📖 Frankfurter, wiener, or hot dog, Average Value ☞ 28 (Low)

📖 Fruit salad— with citrus fruits ☞ 41 (Low)

📖 Fruit salad—no citrus fruits with cream substitute ☞ 46 (Low)

📖 Fruit salad—with cream, no citrus fruits ☞ 48 (Low)

📖 Fruit salad—with mayonnaise ☞ 49 (Low)

📖 Fruit—chocolate covered ☞ 54 (Low)

📖 Italian pie, whitount meat or poultry ☞ 60 (Medium)

📖 Knockwurst ☞ 28 (Low)

📖 Luncheon loaf—with olive, pickle, and/or pimiento ☞ 28 (Low)

📖 Luncheon meat— Average Value ☞ 28 (Low)

📖 Macaroni—creamed, with cheese ☞ 43 (Low)

📖 Macaroni—salad ☞ 45 (Low)

📖 Meat loaf—prepared with beef ☞ 61 (Medium)

📖 Meat loaf—prepared with beef, tomato sauce ☞ 56 (Medium)

📖 Meat loaf—prepared with chicken or turkey ☞ 60 (Medium)

📖 Mettwurst ☞ 28 (Low)

📖 Mortadella ☞ 28 (Low)

📖 Pasta salad ☞ 46 (Low)

📖 Pepper steak ☞ 46 (Low)

📖 Pepperoni ☞ 28 (Low)

📖 Pizza—cheese, NS as to type of crust ☞ 60 (Medium)

📖 Pizza—cheese, thick crust ☞ 60 (Medium)

📖 Pizza—cheese, thin crust ☞ 60 (Medium)

📖 Pizza—cheese, with fruit, thick crust ☞ 60 (Medium)

📖 Pizza—cheese, with vegetables, NS as to type of crust ☞ 49 (Low)

📖 Pizza—cheese, with vegetables, thick crust ☞ 49 (Low)

📖 Pizza—cheese, with vegetables, thin crust ☞ 49 (Low)

📖 Pizza—no cheese, thick crust ☞ 80 (High)

📖 Pizza—with meat and fruit, thick crust ☞ 36 (Low)

📖 Pizza—with meat and fruit, thin crust ☞ 30 (Low)

📖 Pizza—with meat and vegetables, lowfat, thin crust ☞ 30 (Low)

📖 Pizza—with meat and vegetables, NS as to type of crust ☞ 30 (Low)

📖 Pizza—with meat and vegetables, thick crust ☞ 36 (Low)

📖 Pizza—with meat and vegetables, thin crust ☞ 30 (Low)

📖 Pizza—with meat, NS as to type of crust ☞ 30 (Low)

📖 Pizza—with meat, thick crust ☞ 36 (Low)

📖 Pizza—with meat, thin crust ☞ 30 (Low)

📖 Polish sausage ☞ 28 (Low)

📖 Pork roll—cured, fried ☞ 28 (Low)

📖 Potato salad ☞ 66 (Medium)

📖 Potato salad—German style ☞ 68 (Medium)

📖 Potato salad—with egg ☞ 66 (Medium)

Pudding—bread ☞ 62 (Medium)

Pudding—fruit, vanilla wafers ☞ 59 (Medium)

Roast beef sandwich ☞ 70 (High)

Roast beef sandwich—with cheese ☞ 69 (Medium)

Salami—Average Value ☞ 28 (Low)

Salami—beef ☞ 28 (Low)

Salami—dry or hard ☞ 28 (Low)

Salami—soft, cooked ☞ 28 (Low)

Salisbury steak with gravy ☞ 64 (Medium)

Sandwich loaf—luncheon meat ☞ 28 (Low)

Sausage— lowfat, smoked, turkey, pork, and beef ☞ 28 (Low)

Sausage—Average Value ☞ 28 (Low)

Sausage—from fresh, cooked bulk, patty or link, with turkey and pork ☞ 28 (Low)

Sausage—from fresh, pork, bulk, patty or link, cooked ☞ 28 (Low)

Sausage—from fresh, pork, country style, cooked ☞ 28 (Low)

Sausage—Italian ☞ 28 (Low)

Sausage—Pork and Beef ☞ 28 (Low)

Sausage—Pork and Beef brown and serve, cooked ☞ 28 (Low)

Sausage—pork, brown and serve, cooked ☞ 28 (Low)

Sausage—reduced fat, smoked, turkey, pork, and beef ☞ 28 (Low)

Sausage—Smoked link , pork ☞ 28 (Low)

Sausage—Smoked link, pork and beef ☞ 28 (Low)

Sausage—smoked, pork ☞ 28 (Low)

📖 Sausage—smoked, turkey ☛ 28 (Low)

📖 Sausage—Vienna, canned ☛ 28 (Low)

📖 Sausage—Vienna, canned, chicken ☛ 28 (Low)

📖 Scrapple—cooked ☛ 28 (Low)

📖 Soft taco with beef ☛ 30 (Low)

📖 Souse ☛ 28 (Low)

📖 Sweet and sour turkey ☛ 53 (Low)

📖 Taco salad—with beef, cheese, corn chips ☛ 56 (Medium)

📖 Taco—with beans, meat, lettuce, cheese, tomato and salsa ☛ 55 (Low)

📖 Taco—with beef, lettuce and cheese ☛ 68 (Medium)

📖 Taco—with beef, tomato, lettuce, cheese, and salsa ☛ 58 (Medium)

📖 Tamale prepared with meat and/or chicken ☛ 62 (Medium)

📖 Thuringer ☛ 28 (Low)

📖 Turkey bacon—cooked ☛ 50 (Low)

📖 Turkey parmigiana ☛ 79 (High)

📖 Turkey pot pie ☛ 85 (High)

📖 Turkey salad ☛ 41 (Low)

📖 Turkey teriyaki ☛ 57 (Medium)

📖 Turkey with barbecue sauce ☛ 38 (Low)

📖 Turkey with dumplings ☛ 91 (High)

23

RECIPES

🐾 Beef and noodles—with tomato sauce ☞ 40 (Low)

🐾 Beef and vegetables—carrots, broccoli, dark-green leafy, soy-based sauce ☞ 49 (Low)

🐾 Beef stew—with potatoes, tomato sauce ☞ 70 (Medium)

🐾 Beef stroganoff—with noodles ☞ 46 (Low)

🐾 Beef vegetables stew—potatoes, carrots, broccoli, dark-green leafy, tomato sauce ☞ 63 (Medium)

🐾 Beef vegetables stew—potatoes, carrots, broccoli, dark-green leafy ☞ 64 (Medium)

🐾 Beef—sloppy joe without bun ☞ 42 (Low)

🐾 Beef—with barbecue sauce ☞ 38 (Low)

🐾 Beef—with gravy ☞ 71 (High)

🐾 Beef—with tomato sauce ☞ 37 (Low)

🐾 Burrito—beef, with beans, sour cream and cheese ☞ 33 (Low)

Burrito—sausage, cheese, eggs and vegetables ☞ 31 (Low)

Burrito—with beef and beans ☞ 34 (Low)

Burrito—with beef and cheese, whitout beans ☞ 30 (Low)

Burrito—with beef, with beans, and cheese ☞ 34 (Low)

Burrito—with cheese, beans, without meat or poultry ☞ 34 (Low)

Chicken and noodles—no sauce ☞ 40 (Low)

Chicken and noodles—with cream or white sauce ☞ 46 (Low)

Chicken fillet sandwich—broiled, cheese, lettuce, tomato, spread, and bun ☞ 59 (Medium)

Chicken fillet sandwich—broiled, lettuce, tomato, spread and whole-wheat roll ☞ 69 (Medium)

Chicken garden salad—tomato, carrots, other vegetables, no potato, no dressing ☞ 32 (Low)

Chicken or turkey—cacciatore ☞ 61 (Medium)

Chicken or turkey—cordon bleu ☞ 82 (High)

Chicken parmigiana ☞ 79 (High)

Chicken patty sandwich ☞ 67 (Medium)

Chicken pot pie ☞ 85 (High)

Chicken salad ☞ 41 (Low)

Chicken teriyaki ☞ 57 (Medium)

Chicken with barbecue sauce ☞ 38 (Low)

Chicken with dumplings ☞ 91 (High)

Chicken with vegetables—carrots, broccoli, dark-green leafy without sauce ☞ 43 (Low)

Chicken with vegetables—carrots, broccoli, dark-green leafy, with soy-based sauce ☞ 55 (Low)

Chiles rellenos ☞ 35 (Low)

Chili con carne—beans ☞ 34 (Low)

Chili con carne—beans and cheese ☞ 34 (Low)

Chili con carne—beans and rice ☞ 55 (Low)

Chili con carne—beans, macaroni ☞ 41 (Low)

Chili con carne—beans, made with chicken ☞ 34 (Low)

Chili con carne—beans, made with turkey ☞ 34 (Low)

Chili con carne—beans, made with venison/deer ☞ 34 (Low)

Chili con carne—beans, prepared with pork ☞ 34 (Low)

Chili con carne—without beans ☞ 37 (Low)

Fajita with chicken and vegetables ☞ 31 (Low)

Fruit salad— with citrus fruits ☞ 41 (Low)

Fruit salad—no citrus fruits with cream substitute ☞ 46 (Low)

Fruit salad—with cream, no citrus fruits ☞ 48 (Low)

Fruit salad—with mayonnaise ☞ 49 (Low)

Fruit—chocolate covered ☞ 54 (Low)

Macaroni—creamed, with cheese ☞ 43 (Low)

Macaroni—salad ☞ 45 (Low)

Meat loaf—prepared with beef ☞ 61 (Medium)

Meat loaf—prepared with beef, tomato sauce ☞ 56 (Medium)

Meat loaf—prepared with chicken or turkey ☞ 60 (Medium)

Pasta salad ☞ 46 (Low)

Pepper steak ☞ 46 (Low)

Potato salad ☞ 66 (Medium)

Potato salad—German style ☞ 68 (Medium)

Potato salad—with egg ☞ 66 (Medium)

Pudding—bread ☞ 62 (Medium)

Pudding—fruit, vanilla wafers ☞ 59 (Medium)

Roast beef sandwich ☞ 70 (High)

Roast beef sandwich—with cheese ☞ 69 (Medium)

Salisbury steak with gravy ☞ 64 (Medium)

Soft taco with beef ☞ 30 (Low)

Sweet and sour turkey ☞ 53 (Low)

Taco salad—with beef, cheese, corn chips ☞ 56 (Medium)

Taco—with beans, meat, lettuce, cheese, tomato and salsa ☞ 55 (Low)

Taco—with beef, lettuce and cheese ☞ 68 (Medium)

Taco—with beef, tomato, lettuce, cheese, and salsa ☞ 58 (Medium)

Tamale prepared with meat and/or chicken ☞ 62 (Medium)

Turkey parmigiana ☞ 79 (High)

Turkey pot pie ☞ 85 (High)

Turkey salad ☞ 41 (Low)

Turkey teriyaki ☞ 57 (Medium)

Turkey with barbecue sauce ☞ 38 (Low)

Turkey with dumplings ☞ 91 (High)

24

SNACK FOODS AND CONFECTIONERY

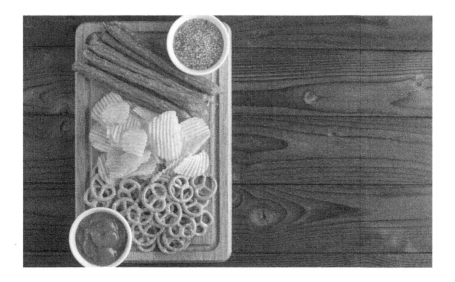

This extensive list comprises 4000+ brand-name and generic foods with their respective glycemic index values. Data were compiled from various authoritative sources and some GI values were calculated as the mean of up to five studies.

◎ Bagel chip ☛ 72 (High)

◎ Biscuit dough, fried ☛ 66 (Medium)

◎ Biscuit— baking powder / buttermilk, commercially baked ☛ 92 (High)

◎ Biscuit— baking powder / buttermilk, made from mix ☛ 92 (High)

◎ Biscuit— baking powder / buttermilk, made from refrigerated dough ☛ 92 (High)

◎ Biscuit— baking powder / buttermilk, made from refrigerated dough, lowfat ☛ 92 (High)

◎ Biscuit— baking powder / buttermilk, NS as to made from mix, refrigerated dough, or home recipe ☛ 92 (High)

◎ Biscuit— baking powder / buttermilk, prepared from home recipe ☛ 92 (High)

◎ Bread stick—hard, whole wheat ☛ 83 (High)

◎ Bread sticks, hard ☛ 70 (High)

◎ Cashew butter ☛ 22 (Low)

◎ Cashew nuts—average ☛ 22 (Low)

◎ Cashew nuts—dry roasted ☛ 22 (Low)

◎ Cashew nuts—roasted, with salt ☛ 22 (Low)

◎ Cashew nuts—roasted, without salt ☛ 22 (Low)

◎ Chocolate— milk, plain ☛ 43 (Low)

◎ Chocolate— milk, with almonds ☛ 43 (Low)

◎ Chocolate— milk, with cereal ☛ 43 (Low)

◎ Chocolate— milk, with fruit and nuts ☛ 43 (Low)

◎ Chocolate— milk, with nuts, not almond or peanuts ☛ 43 (Low)

Chocolate— milk, with peanuts ☞ 43 (Low)

Chocolate— semi-sweet morsel ☞ 43 (Low)

Chocolate— sweet or dark ☞ 43 (Low)

Chocolate— white ☞ 44 (Low)

Chocolate— white, with almonds ☞ 44 (Low)

Chocolate— white, with cereal ☞ 44 (Low)

Coconut candy—chocolate covered ☞ 43 (Low)

Cookie— almond ☞ 64 (Medium)

Cookie— batter or dough, raw, not chocolate ☞ 64 (Medium)

Cookie— brownie, diet, NS as to icing ☞ 51 (Low)

Cookie— brownie, fat free, cholesterol free, with icing ☞ 51 (Low)

Cookie— brownie, fat free, without icing ☞ 51 (Low)

Cookie— brownie, lowfat, with icing ☞ 51 (Low)

Cookie— brownie, lowfat, without icing ☞ 51 (Low)

Cookie— brownie, with cream cheese filling, without icing ☞ 51 (Low)

Cookie— brownie, with icing ☞ 51 (Low)

Cookie— brownie, with peanut butter fudge icing ☞ 51 (Low)

Cookie— brownie, without icing ☞ 51 (Low)

Cookie— butter or sugar cookie ☞ 55 (Low)

Cookie— butter or sugar, with chocolate icing or filling ☞ 49 (Low)

Cookie— butterscotch chip ☞ 64 (Medium)

Cookie— butterscotch, brownie ☞ 53 (Low)

◎ Cookie— chocolate and vanilla sandwich ☛ 49 (Low)

◎ Cookie— chocolate chip ☛ 49 (Low)

◎ Cookie— chocolate chip sandwich ☛ 49 (Low)

◎ Cookie— chocolate chip, purchased at a bakery ☛ 49 (Low)

◎ Cookie— chocolate chip, reduced fat ☛ 42 (Low)

◎ Cookie— chocolate chip, with raisins ☛ 49 (Low)

◎ Cookie— chocolate fudge, with nuts ☛ 49 (Low)

◎ Cookie— chocolate sandwich, reduced fat ☛ 42 (Low)

◎ Cookie— chocolate-covered, chocolate sandwich ☛ 49 (Low)

◎ Cookie— Chocolate— chocolate sandwich or chocolate-coated or striped ☛ 49 (Low)

◎ Cookie— Chocolate— sandwich, with extra filling ☛ 49 (Low)

◎ Cookie— Chocolate— with chocolate filling or coating, fat free ☛ 42 (Low)

◎ Cookie— date bar ☛ 51 (Low)

◎ Cookie— dietetic, NFS ☛ 58 (Medium)

◎ Cookie— dietetic, oatmeal with raisins ☛ 58 (Medium)

◎ Cookie— dietetic, sugar or plain ☛ 58 (Medium)

◎ Cookie— fig bar ☛ 51 (Low)

◎ Cookie— fig bar, fat free ☛ 51 (Low)

◎ Cookie— fortune ☛ 77 (High)

◎ Cookie— fruit-filled bar ☛ 51 (Low)

◎ Cookie— fruit-filled bar, fat free ☛ 51 (Low)

◎ Cookie— gingersnaps ☛ 77 (High)

Cookie— graham cracker sandwich with chocolate ☛ 74 (High)

Cookie— oatmeal ☛ 54 (Low)

Cookie— oatmeal sandwich, with creme filling ☛ 54 (Low)

Cookie— oatmeal, fat free, with raisins ☛ 54 (Low)

Cookie— oatmeal, reduced fat, with raisins ☛ 54 (Low)

Cookie— oatmeal, with chocolate chips ☛ 54 (Low)

Cookie— oatmeal, with fruit filling ☛ 54 (Low)

Cookie— oatmeal, with raisins ☛ 54 (Low)

Cookie— peanut butter ☛ 64 (Medium)

Cookie— rich, all Chocolate— with chocolate chips ☛ 49 (Low)

Cookie— rich, with chocolate filling ☛ 49 (Low)

Cookie— shortbread ☛ 64 (Medium)

Cookie— shortbread, reduced fat ☛ 64 (Medium)

Cookie— shortbread, with chocolate filling ☛ 57 (Medium)

Cookie— tea, Japanese ☛ 55 (Low)

Cookie— vanilla sandwich ☛ 77 (High)

Cookie— vanilla sandwich, reduced fat ☛ 77 (High)

Cookie— vanilla wafer ☛ 77 (High)

Cookie— vanilla wafer, reduced fat ☛ 77 (High)

Cookie— vanilla waffle creme ☛ 77 (High)

Cookie— vanilla with caramel, coconut, and chocolate coating ☛ 63 (Medium)

Cookie—Average value ☛ 57 (Medium)

Cracker—100% whole wheat ☛ 67 (Medium)

Cracker—100% whole wheat, low sodium ☞ 67 (Medium)

Cracker—100% whole wheat, reduced fat ☞ 67 (Medium)

Cracker—animal ☞ 65 (Medium)

Cracker—cheese ☞ 55 (Low)

Cracker—cheese, low sodium ☞ 55 (Low)

Cracker—cheese, reduced fat ☞ 55 (Low)

Cracker—graham, sugar-honey coated, cinnamon crisps ☞ 74 (High)

Cracker—sandwich-type, peanut butter filled ☞ 59 (Medium)

Cracker—snack ☞ 55 (Low)

Cracker—snack, fat free ☞ 55 (Low)

Cracker—snack, low sodium ☞ 55 (Low)

Cracker—snack, lowfat, low sodium ☞ 55 (Low)

Cracker—snack, reduced fat ☞ 55 (Low)

Crackers—graham ☞ 74 (High)

Crackers—graham, chocolate covered ☞ 74 (High)

Crackers—graham, fat free ☞ 74 (High)

Crackers—graham, higher fat ☞ 74 (High)

Crackers—graham, lowfat ☞ 74 (High)

Crackers—matzo ☞ 71 (High)

Crackers—matzo, low sodium ☞ 71 (High)

Crackers—milk ☞ 55 (Low)

Crackers—NS as to sweet or nonsweet ☞ 74 (High)

Crackers—oyster ☞ 71 (High)

◎ Crackers—saltine ☛ 74 (High)

◎ Crackers—saltine, fat free, low sodium ☛ 74 (High)

◎ Crackers—saltine, low sodium ☛ 74 (High)

◎ Crackers—saltine, whole wheat ☛ 67 (Medium)

◎ Crackers—toast thins ☛ 70 (High)

◎ Crackers—toast thins, low sodium ☛ 70 (High)

◎ Crackers—water biscuits ☛ 71 (High)

◎ Crackers—wheat ☛ 67 (Medium)

◎ Crackers—wheat, reduced fat ☛ 67 (Medium)

◎ Crispbread—rye, no added fat ☛ 64 (Medium)

◎ Crispbread—wheat or rye, extra crispy ☛ 64 (Medium)

◎ Crispbread—wheat, no added fat ☛ 55 (Low)

◎ Fondant—chocolate covered ☛ 43 (Low)

◎ Fruit butter ☛ 51 (Low)

◎ Fruit leather ☛ 99 (High)

◎ Granola bar—chocolate-coated ☛ 62 (Medium)

◎ Granola bar—coated without chocolate coating ☛ 51 (Low)

◎ Granola bar—high fiber, coated without coating ☛ 51 (Low)

◎ Granola bar—nonfat ☛ 61 (Medium)

◎ Granola bar—oats, fruit and nuts, lowfat ☛ 61 (Medium)

◎ Granola bar—oats, sugar, raisins, coconut ☛ 61 (Medium)

◎ Granola bar—Peanuts—oats, sugar, wheat germ ☛ 61 (Medium)

◎ Granola bar—with coconut, chocolate-coated ☛ 62 (Medium)

◎ Granola bar—with nuts ☛ 62 (Medium)

◎ Granola bar—with rice cereal ☛ 63 (Medium)

◎ Gumdrops ☛ 78 (High)

◎ Hard candy ☛ 70 (High)

◎ Jams, or marmalades—dietetic, all flavors ☛ 55 (Low)

◎ Jams, preserves, marmalades, low sugar (all flavors) ☛ 55 (Low)

◎ Jelly—diet, sweetened with artificial sweetener ☛ 55 (Low)

◎ Jelly—reduced sugar, all flavors ☛ 55 (Low)

◎ Licorice ☛ 78 (High)

◎ Peanut butter ☛ 14 (Low)

◎ Peanut butter—low sodium ☛ 14 (Low)

◎ Peanut butter—reduced fat ☛ 14 (Low)

◎ Peanut butter—reduced sodium ☛ 14 (Low)

◎ Peanuts—average value ☛ 14 (Low)

◎ Peanuts—boiled ☛ 14 (Low)

◎ Peanuts—dry roasted, salted ☛ 14 (Low)

◎ Peanuts—dry roasted, without salt ☛ 14 (Low)

◎ Peanuts—honey-roasted ☛ 14 (Low)

◎ Peanuts—roasted, salted ☛ 14 (Low)

◎ Peanuts—roasted, without salt ☛ 14 (Low)

◎ Pecans ☛ 20 (Low)

◎ Planters Peanut Bar ☛ 23 (Low)

◎ Popcorn—air-popped (no butter or no oil added) ☛ 72 (High)

- Popcorn—air-popped, buttered ☛ 72 (High)

- Popcorn—flavored ☛ 72 (High)

- Popcorn—popped in oil, buttered ☛ 72 (High)

- Popcorn—popped in oil, lowfat ☛ 72 (High)

- Popcorn—popped in oil, lowfat, low sodium ☛ 72 (High)

- Popcorn—popped in oil, unbuttered ☛ 72 (High)

- Popcorn—popped in oil, unsalted ☛ 72 (High)

- Popcorn—with cheese ☛ 72 (High)

- Pretzels—average value ☛ 83 (High)

- Pretzels—hard ☛ 83 (High)

- Pretzels—hard, unsalted ☛ 83 (High)

- Pretzels—oatbran, hard ☛ 83 (High)

- Pretzels—soft ☛ 83 (High)

- Puffed rice cake ☛ 78 (High)

- Scone ☛ 92 (High)

- Scone, with fruit ☛ 92 (High)

- Skittles ☛ 70 (High)

- Sunflower seeds, unroasted ☛ 20 (Low)

- Walnuts ☛ 20 (Low)

- White potato skins, chips ☛ 54 (Low)

- White potato—chips ☛ 54 (Low)

- White potato—chips, fat free ☛ 54 (Low)

- White potato—chips, reduced fat ☛ 54 (Low)

⊙ White potato—chips, reduced fat and reduced sodium ☞ 54 (Low)

⊙ White potato—chips, restructured ☞ 54 (Low)

⊙ White potato—chips, unsalted ☞ 54 (Low)

⊙ White potato—chips, unsalted, reduced fat ☞ 54 (Low)

⊙ White potato—sticks ☞ 54 (Low)

25

SOUPS, PASTA AND NOODLES

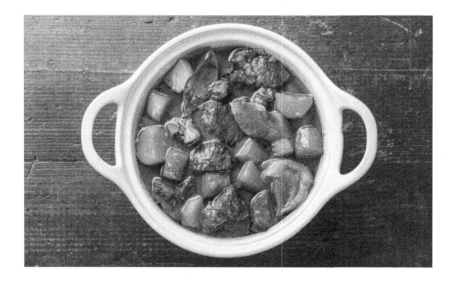

What is the serving size?

The typical serving sizes for low GI Soups, Pasta and Noodles are equivalent to:

- 1 cup vegetable soup

- ½ cup of cooked cereal, pasta, or other cooked grain
- ⅓ cup of cooked rice, and other small grains

For moderate GI Soups, Pasta and Noodles reduce the serving by 1/3

How Much a Day?

Up to 8 servings per day provided you respect your calorie deficit in your overall daily intake.

———

🍲 Asparagus soup—made with milk or water ☛ 27 (Low)

🍲 Asparagus soup—prepared with milk ☛ 27 (Low)

🍲 Barley soup ☛ 25 (Low)

🍲 Bean and ham soup—chunky style ☛ 64 (Medium)

🍲 Bean and ham soup—home recipe ☛ 64 (Medium)

🍲 Bean and rice soup ☛ 42.2 (Low)

🍲 Bean soup—average ☛ 64 (Medium)

🍲 Bean soup—home recipe ☛ 64 (Medium)

🍲 Bean soup—mixed beans ☛ 64 (Medium)

🍲 Bean soup—with bacon or pork ☛ 64 (Medium)

🍲 Bean soup—with macaroni ☛ 37.8 (Low)

🍲 Bean soup—with macaroni and meat ☛ 38.3 (Low)

🍲 Bean soup—with vegetables and rice ☛ 55.3 (Medium)

🍲 Beef and rice noodle soup ☛ 53 (Low)

🍲 Beef noodle soup ☛ 42 (Low)

🍲 Beef noodle soup—home recipe ☛ 42 (Low)

- Beef noodle soup—Sopa de carne y fideos ☞ 42 (Low)

- Beef pot pie ☞ 45 (Low)

- Beef rice soup ☞ 64 (Low)

- Beef stroganoff soup—chunky style ☞ 42 (Low)

- Beef stroganoff—with noodles ☞ 46 (Low)

- Beef vegetable soup—Sopa caldo de Res ☞ 38 (Low)

- Beef vegetable soup—with noodles, stew type, chunky style ☞ 40 (Low)

- Beef vegetable soup—with potato, stew type ☞ 44 (Low)

- Beef vegetable soup—with rice, stew type, chunky style ☞ 51 (Low)

- Beef, rice, and vegetables soup —not carrots, not broccoli ☞ 49.1 (Low)

- Beef, rice, and vegetables soup—with carrots, broccoli ☞ 47.4 (Low)

- Black bean soup ☞ 64 (Medium)

- Broccoli cheese soup—prepared with milk ☞ 27 (Low)

- Broccoli soup ☞ 27 (Low)

- Carrot soup—prepared with milk ☞ 37 (Low)

- Cauliflower soup—prepared with milk ☞ 27 (Low)

- Celery soup—made with milk or water, average value ☞ 27 (Low)

- Celery soup—prepared with milk ☞ 27 (Low)

- Celery soup—prepared with water ☞ 27 (Low)

- Cheddar cheese soup ☞ 27 (Low)

- Chicken and mushroom soup—prepared with milk ☞ 27 (Low)

🍲 Chicken gumbo soup ☞ 38 (Low)

🍲 Chicken noodle soup ☞ 42 (Low)

🍲 Chicken noodle soup—canned ☞ 42 (Low)

🍲 Chicken noodle soup—canned ☞ 42 (Low)

🍲 Chicken noodle soup—chunky style ☞ 40 (Low)

🍲 Chicken noodle soup—cream of ☞ 34.5 (Low)

🍲 Chicken noodle soup—home recipe ☞ 42 (Low)

🍲 Chicken or turkey rice soup—home recipe ☞ 64 (Medium)

🍲 Chicken or turkey soup—canned, prepared with milk ☞ 27 (Low)

🍲 Chicken or turkey soup—canned, prepared with water ☞ 27 (Low)

🍲 Chicken or turkey soup—canned, undiluted ☞ 27 (Low)

🍲 Chicken or turkey soup—prepared with milk ☞ 27 (Low)

🍲 Chicken or turkey soup—prepared with water ☞ 27 (Low)

🍲 Chicken or turkey soup—with milk or water, average value ☞ 27 (Low)

🍲 Chicken or turkey vegetable soup—home recipe ☞ 38 (Low)

🍲 Chicken or turkey vegetable soup—stew type ☞ 38 (Low)

🍲 Chicken rice soup ☞ 64 (Medium)

🍲 Chicken rice soup—canned ☞ 64 (Medium)

🍲 Chicken rice soup—Sopa de pollo con arroz ☞ 64 (Medium)

🍲 Chicken soup ☞ 42 (Low)

🍲 Chicken soup—with noodles and potatoes ☞ 57 (Medium)

🍲 Chicken soup—with vegetables, Oriental style ☞ 38 (Low)

🍲 Chicken vegetable soup—with noodles, chunky style ☞ 40 (Low)

- Chicken vegetable soup—with potato, cheese, chunky style ☞ 44 (Low)

- Chicken vegetable soup—with rice, stew type ☞ 51 (Low)

- Chickpea soup ☞ 64 (Low)

- Chili beef soup ☞ 51 (Low)

- Chili beef soup—chunky style ☞ 51 (Low)

- Corn soup—prepared with milk ☞ 40.5 (Low)

- Corn soup—prepared with water ☞ 40.5 (Low)

- Crab soup—prepared with milk ☞ 27 (Low)

- Crab soup—tomato-base ☞ 38 (Low)

- Cucumber soup—prepared with milk ☞ 27 (Low)

- Dark-green leafy vegetable soup ☞ 38 (Low)

- Dark-green leafy vegetable soup, meatless ☞ 38 (Low)

- Ham soup— with chunky pea ☞ 66 (Medium)

- Ham, potato, and rice soup ☞ 51 (Low)

- Instant soup rice ☞ 64 (Low)

- Instant soup, noodle ☞ 42 (Low)

- Instant soup, noodle—with chicken, egg, or shrimp ☞ 42 (Low)

- Leek soup—prepared with milk ☞ 27 (Low)

- Lentil soup ☞ 44 (Low)

- Lima bean soup ☞ 60 (Medium)

- Macaroni and potato soup ☞ 62.5 (Medium)

- Meat and corn hominy soup ☞ 40 (Low)

- Meatball soup—Sopa de Albondigas ☞ 38 (Low)

Minestrone soup—canned ☞ 39 (Low)

Minestrone soup—home recipe ☞ 39 (Low)

Mushroom soup—average value ☞ 27 (Low)

Mushroom soup—canned, made with milk, ☞ 27 (Low)

Mushroom soup—cream of, with milk ☞ 27 (Low)

Mushroom soup—made with water, cream of ☞ 27 (Low)

Mushroom soup—prepared with water ☞ 27 (Low)

Mushroom soup—undiluted ☞ 27 (Low)

Noodle and potato soup ☞ 42 (Low)

Noodle soup with vegetable—Oriental style ☞ 40 (Low)

Noodle soup—average value ☞ 42 (Low)

Noodle soup—with fish ball, and/or shrimp, and dark green leafy vegetable ☞ 42 (Low)

Oxtail soup ☞ 38 (Low)

Pasta salad—macaroni or noodles, and vegetables ☞ 45.6 (Low)

Pasta—canned, with tomato sauce and cheese ☞ 40 (Low)

Pasta—canned, with tomato sauce and meatballs ☞ 52 (Low)

Pasta—cooked, corn-based, average value ☞ 78 (High)

Pasta—cooked, corn-based, with fat ☞ 78 (High)

Pasta—with carbonara sauce ☞ 42 (Low)

Pasta—with cheese and meat sauce ☞ 52 (Low)

Pasta—with meat sauce ☞ 52 (Low)

Pasta—without meat or poultry, with cheese and tomato sauce ☞ 40 (Low)

🍲 Pasta—without meat or poultry, with tomato sauce ☞ 40 (Low)

🍲 Pea soup—canned, made with water ☞ 66 (Medium)

🍲 Pea soup—common ☞ 66 (Medium)

🍲 Pea soup—instant type ☞ 66 (Medium)

🍲 Pea soup—made with mill ☞ 46.5 (Low)

🍲 Pea soup—made with water ☞ 66 (Medium)

🍲 Pork and rice soup—stew type / chunky style ☞ 51 (Low)

🍲 Pork vegetable soup—with noodles, stew type /chunky style ☞ 40 (Low)

🍲 Pork with vegetable soup—no carrots, no dark-green leafy ☞ 38 (Low)

🍲 Pork, vegetable soup—with potatoes /stew type ☞ 38 (Low)

🍲 Potato and cheese soup ☞ 53.9 (Low)

🍲 Potato soup— prepared with milk ☞ 49.5 (Low)

🍲 Potato soup—average value ☞ 49.5 (Low)

🍲 Potato soup—made with water ☞ 49.5 (Low)

🍲 Rice and potato soup—Puerto Rican style ☞ 64 (Medium)

🍲 Rice soup—average value ☞ 64 (Medium)

🍲 Salmon soup—cream style ☞ 27 (Low)

🍲 Seasoned shredded soup with meat ☞ 50 (Low)

🍲 Shrimp soup—prepared with milk ☞ 27 (Low)

🍲 Soup—average value ☞ 38 (Low)

🍲 Soup—mostly noodles ☞ 42 (Low)

🍲 Soybean soup—made with milk ☞ 43.5 (Low)

Soybean soup—miso broth ☞ 29.2 (Low)

Spaghetti—cooked, average value ☞ 42 (Low)

Spaghetti—cooked, with fat ☞ 42 (Low)

Spaghetti—whole wheat spaghetti, with tomato sauce and meat ☞ 52 (Low)

Spaghetti—with clam sauce ☞ 40 (Low)

Spaghetti—with red clam sauce ☞ 40 (Low)

Spaghetti—with tomato sauce and hot dogs ☞ 52 (Low)

Spaghetti—with tomato sauce and meatballs ☞ 52 (Low)

Spaghetti—with tomato sauce and poultry ☞ 52 (Low)

Spaghetti—with white clam sauce ☞ 42 (Low)

Spaghetti—without meat or poultry, tomato sauce ☞ 40 (Low)

Spaghetti,—cooked, whitout fat ☞ 42 (Low)

Split pea soup ☞ 60 (Medium)

Split pea soup—canned ☞ 60 (Medium)

Split peas soup—with ham ☞ 60 (Medium)

Split peas soup—with ham, canned ☞ 60 (Medium)

Tomato beef noodle soup—made with water ☞ 40 (Low)

Tomato beef soup—made with water ☞ 38 (Low)

Tomato noodle soup—made with water ☞ 40 (Low)

Tomato soup—average value ☞ 38 (Low)

Tomato soup—canned ☞ 38 (Low)

Tomato soup—canned, undiluted ☞ 38 (Low)

Tomato soup—instant type, made with water ☞ 38 (Low)

Tomato soup—made with water ☞ 38 (Low)

Tomato soup—prepared with milk ☞ 35.7 (Low)

Tomato vegetable soup—made with water ☞ 38 (Low)

Tomato vegetable soup—with noodles, made with water ☞ 40 (Low)

Turkey noodle soup ☞ 42 (Low)

Turkey noodle soup—home recipe ☞ 42 (Low)

Vegetable bean soup—ready-to-serve or prepared with water ☞ 39 (Low)

Vegetable beef soup with rice—home recipe ☞ 51 (Low)

Vegetable beef soup with rice—ready-to-serve or prepared with water ☞ 51 (Low)

Vegetable beef soup—canned, undiluted ☞ 38 (Low)

Vegetable beef soup—chunky style ☞ 38 (Low)

Vegetable beef soup—home recipe ☞ 38 (Low)

Vegetable beef soup—home recipe, with noodles or pasta ☞ 40 (Low)

Vegetable beef soup—prepared with water ☞ 38 (Low)

Vegetable chicken noodle soup—prepared with water ☞ 40 (Low)

Vegetable chicken or turkey soup—made with water ☞ 38 (Low)

Vegetable chicken rice soup—with water or ready-to-serve ☞ 51 (Low)

Vegetable chicken soup—canned, prepared with water ☞ 38 (Low)

Vegetable noodle soup—canned, water or ready-to-serve ☞ 40 (Low)

🍲 Vegetable noodle soup—home recipe ☞ 40 (Low)

🍲 Vegetable noodle soup—with water ☞ 40 (Low)

🍲 Vegetable rice soup—prepared with water ☞ 51 (Low)

🍲 Vegetable soup—canned, low sodium, water ☞ 38 (Low)

🍲 Vegetable soup—canned, undiluted ☞ 38 (Low)

🍲 Vegetable soup—chunky style ☞ 38 (Low)

🍲 Vegetable soup—home recipe ☞ 38 (Low)

🍲 Vegetable soup—made from dry mix ☞ 38 (Low)

🍲 Vegetable soup—made with water or ready-to-serve ☞ 38 (Low)

🍲 Vegetable soup—prepared with dry mix, low sodium, water ☞ 32.5 (Low)

🍲 Vegetable soup—prepared with milk ☞ 32.5 (Low)

🍲 Vegetable soup—with chicken broth ☞ 38 (Low)

🍲 Vegetable soup—with pasta, chunky style ☞ 40 (Low)

🍲 Vegetarian vegetable soup—made with water ☞ 38 (Low)

🍲 Zucchini soup—made with milk ☞ 27 (Low)

26

VEGETABLES

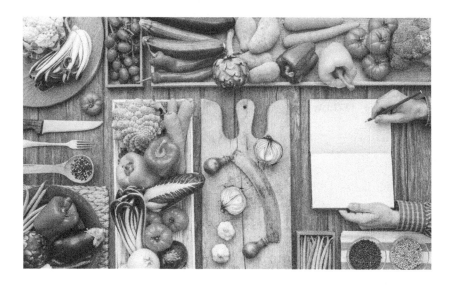

What is the serving size?

The typical serving size for low GI vegetables and vegetables juices can be expressed as

- 1 cup raw or salad vegetables

- 1/2 cup cooked or canned vegetables
- 3/4 cup (6oz) vegetable juice homemade and unsweetened

For moderate GI vegetables and vegetables juices reduce the serving by 1/3

How Much a Day?

Up to 10 servings per day

Alfalfa sprouts, raw ☞ 32 (Low)

Algae, dried ☞ 32 (Low)

Apple, pickled ☞ 38 (Low)

Artichoke— globe (French), cooked, from canned, Not Specified as to with fat ☞ 32 (Low)

Artichoke— globe (French), cooked, from fresh, Not Specified as to with fat ☞ 32 (Low)

Artichoke— globe (French), cooked, from fresh, with fat ☞ 32 (Low)

Artichoke— globe (French), cooked, from fresh, without fat ☞ 32 (Low)

Artichoke— globe (French), cooked, from frozen, Not Specified as to with fat ☞ 32 (Low)

Artichoke— globe (French), cooked, Not Specified as to form, Not Specified as to with fat ☞ 32 (Low)

Artichoke— globe (French), cooked, Not Specified as to form, without fat ☞ 32 (Low)

Artichoke— Jerusalem, raw ☞ 32 (Low)

Artichoke— salad in oil ☞ 32 (Low)

Asparagus— cooked, from canned, Not Specified as to with fat ☞ 32 (Low)

Asparagus— cooked, from canned, with fat ☞ 32 (Low)

Asparagus— cooked, from canned, without fat ☞ 32 (Low)

Asparagus— cooked, from fresh, Not Specified as to with fat ☞ 32 (Low)

Asparagus— cooked, from fresh, with fat ☞ 32 (Low)

Asparagus— cooked, from fresh, without fat ☞ 32 (Low)

Asparagus— cooked, from frozen, with fat ☞ 32 (Low)

Asparagus— cooked, from frozen, without fat ☞ 32 (Low)

Asparagus— cooked, Not Specified as to form, Not Specified as to with fat ☞ 32 (Low)

Asparagus— cooked, Not Specified as to form, with fat ☞ 32 (Low)

Asparagus— cooked, Not Specified as to form, without fat ☞ 32 (Low)

Asparagus— from canned, creamed or with cheese sauce ☞ 28 (Low)

Asparagus— from fresh, creamed or with cheese sauce ☞ 29 (Low)

Asparagus— raw ☞ 32 (Low)

Bamboo shoots—cooked, with fat ☞ 32 (Low)

Bamboo shoots—cooked, without fat ☞ 32 (Low)

Bean sprouts— cooked, from canned, with fat ☞ 32 (Low)

Bean sprouts— cooked, from canned, without fat ☞ 32 (Low)

● Bean sprouts— cooked, from fresh, Not Specified as to with fat ☞ 32 (Low)

● Bean sprouts— cooked, from fresh, with fat ☞ 32 (Low)

● Bean sprouts— cooked, from fresh, without fat ☞ 32 (Low)

● Bean sprouts— cooked, Not Specified as to form, Not Specified as to with fat ☞ 32 (Low)

● Bean sprouts— cooked, Not Specified as to form, with fat ☞ 32 (Low)

● Bean sprouts— raw (soybean or mung) ☞ 32 (Low)

● BeaNot Specified, green string—with tomatoes, cooked, without fat ☞ 35 (Low)

● BeaNot Specified, green—and potatoes, cooked, without fat ☞ 63 (Medium)

● BeaNot Specified, green—with pinto beaNot Specified, cooked, without fat ☞ 38 (Low)

● Beet greeNot Specified—raw ☞ 32 (Low)

● Beets— cooked, from canned, Not Specified as to with fat ☞ 64 (Medium)

● Beets— cooked, from canned, with fat ☞ 64 (Medium)

● Beets— cooked, from canned, without fat ☞ 64 (Medium)

● Beets— cooked, from fresh, Not Specified as to with fat ☞ 64 (Medium)

● Beets— cooked, from fresh, without fat ☞ 64 (Medium)

● Beets— cooked, Not Specified as to form, Not Specified as to with fat ☞ 64 (Medium)

● Beets— cooked, Not Specified as to form, with fat ☞ 64 (Medium)

Beets— cooked, Not Specified as to form, without fat ☞ 64 (Medium)

Beets— pickled ☞ 66 (Medium)

Beets— raw ☞ 64 (Medium)

Beets—with Harvard sauce ☞ 66 (Medium)

Bitter melon—cooked, without fat ☞ 32 (Low)

Breadfruit—cooked, without fat ☞ 68 (Medium)

Broccoflower—cooked, without fat ☞ 32 (Low)

Broccoli—cooked, from fresh, without fat ☞ 32 (Low)

Broccoli—cooked, from frozen, without fat ☞ 32 (Low)

Broccoli—cooked, Not Specified as to form, without fat ☞ 32 (Low)

Broccoli—raw ☞ 32 (Low)

Brussels sprouts—cooked, from fresh, without fat ☞ 32 (Low)

Brussels sprouts—cooked, from frozen, without fat ☞ 32 (Low)

Brussels sprouts—cooked, Not Specified as to form, without fat ☞ 32 (Low)

Brussels sprouts—raw ☞ 32 (Low)

Cabbage—Chinese, cooked, Not Specified as to with fat ☞ 32 (Low)

Cabbage—Chinese, cooked, with fat ☞ 32 (Low)

Cabbage—Chinese, cooked, without fat ☞ 32 (Low)

Cabbage—Chinese, raw ☞ 32 (Low)

Cabbage—Chinese, salad, with dressing ☞ 32 (Low)

Cabbage—fresh, pickled, Japanese style ☞ 32 (Low)

● Cabbage—green, cooked, Not Specified as to with fat ☞ 32 (Low)

● Cabbage—green, cooked, with fat ☞ 32 (Low)

● Cabbage—green, cooked, without fat ☞ 32 (Low)

● Cabbage—green, raw ☞ 32 (Low)

● Cabbage—Kim Chee style ☞ 32 (Low)

● Cabbage—red, cooked, Not Specified as to with fat ☞ 32 (Low)

● Cabbage—red, cooked, with fat ☞ 32 (Low)

● Cabbage—red, cooked, without fat ☞ 32 (Low)

● Cabbage—red, pickled ☞ 32 (Low)

● Cabbage—red, raw ☞ 32 (Low)

● Cactus—cooked, Not Specified as to with fat ☞ 7 (Low)

● Cactus—cooked, with fat ☞ 7 (Low)

● Cactus—cooked, without fat ☞ 7 (Low)

● Cactus—raw ☞ 7 (Low)

● Calabaza (Spanish pumpkin), cooked ☞ 75 (High)

● Carrots—canned, low sodium, without fat ☞ 47 (Low)

● Carrots—cooked, from canned, without fat ☞ 47 (Low)

● Carrots—cooked, from fresh, without fat ☞ 47 (Low)

● Carrots—cooked, from frozen, without fat ☞ 47 (Low)

● Carrots—cooked, Not Specified as to form, without fat ☞ 47 (Low)

● Carrots—raw ☞ 16 (Low)

● Cassava bread ☞ 56 (Medium)

● Cassava—cooked, Not Specified as to with fat ☞ 46 (Low)

- Cassava—cooked, without fat ☞ 46 (Low)

- Cauliflower—cooked, from fresh, without fat ☞ 32 (Low)

- Cauliflower—cooked, from frozen, without fat ☞ 32 (Low)

- Cauliflower—cooked, Not Specified as to form, without fat ☞ 32 (Low)

- Cauliflower—pickled ☞ 32 (Low)

- Cauliflower—raw ☞ 32 (Low)

- Celery juice ☞ 32 (Low)

- Celery—cooked, Not Specified as to with fat ☞ 32 (Low)

- Celery—cooked, with fat ☞ 32 (Low)

- Celery—cooked, without fat ☞ 32 (Low)

- Celery—raw ☞ 32 (Low)

- Chard, cooked, without fat ☞ 32 (Low)

- Chives—raw ☞ 32 (Low)

- Christophine—cooked, without fat ☞ 32 (Low)

- Cilantro—raw ☞ 32 (Low)

- Cocktail sauce ☞ 38 (Low)

- Coleslaw, with dressing ☞ 44 (Low)

- Collards—cooked, from canned, without fat ☞ 32 (Low)

- Collards—cooked, from fresh, without fat ☞ 32 (Low)

- Collards, cooked, from frozen, without fat ☞ 32 (Low)

- Corn relish ☞ 54 (Low)

- Corn—with Pepper— cooked, without fat ☞ 54 (Low)

Cucumber salad—made with Cucumber—oil, and vinegar ☞ 32 (Low)

Cucumber salad—with creamy dressing ☞ 32 (Low)

Cucumber—cooked, Not Specified as to with fat ☞ 32 (Low)

Cucumber—cooked, with fat ☞ 32 (Low)

Cucumber—cooked, without fat ☞ 32 (Low)

Cucumber—pickles, dill ☞ 32 (Low)

Cucumber—pickles, dill, reduced salt ☞ 32 (Low)

Cucumber—pickles, fresh ☞ 32 (Low)

Cucumber—pickles, relish ☞ 32 (Low)

Cucumber—raw ☞ 32 (Low)

Cucumber,pickles, sour ☞ 32 (Low)

Cucumber,pickles, sweet ☞ 32 (Low)

Dandelion greeNot Specified—cooked, without fat ☞ 32 (Low)

Dandelion greeNot Specified—raw ☞ 32 (Low)

Dasheen—boiled ☞ 32 (Low)

Dumpling—potato- or cheese-filled ☞ 52 (Low)

Eggplant—cooked, Not Specified as to with fat ☞ 32 (Low)

Eggplant—cooked, tomato sauce, without fat ☞ 35 (Low)

Eggplant—cooked, with fat ☞ 32 (Low)

Eggplant—cooked, without fat ☞ 32 (Low)

Eggplant—pickled ☞ 32 (Low)

Endive—raw ☞ 32 (Low)

Escarole—cooked, without fat ☞ 32 (Low)

Garlic—cooked ☛ 32 (Low)

Garlic—raw ☛ 32 (Low)

GreeNot Specified—cooked, from canned, without fat ☛ 32 (Low)

GreeNot Specified—cooked, from fresh, without fat ☛ 32 (Low)

Jicama—raw ☛ 32 (Low)

Kale—cooked, from fresh, without fat ☛ 32 (Low)

Leek—raw ☛ 32 (Low)

Lettuce—arugula, raw ☛ 32 (Low)

Lettuce—Boston, raw ☛ 32 (Low)

Lettuce—cooked, without fat ☛ 32 (Low)

Lettuce—raw ☛ 32 (Low)

Lotus root—cooked, without fat ☛ 32 (Low)

Mixed salad—greeNot Specified, raw ☛ 32 (Low)

Mixed vegetables—corn, lima carrots, beaNot Specified, peas, and green beaNot Specified, without fat ☛ 43 (Low)

Mixed vegetables—from canned, corn, carrots, lima beaNot Specified, peas, and green beaNot Specified, cooked, without fat ☛ 43 (Low)

Mixed vegetables—from corn, carrots, lima beaNot Specified, peas, and green beaNot Specified, without fat ☛ 43 (Low)

Mixed vegetables—from frozen, corn, lima beaNot Specified, carrots, peas, and green beaNot Specified, without fat ☛ 43 (Low)

Mushroom—Oriental, cooked, from dried ☛ 32 (Low)

Mushrooms—cooked, from canned, Not Specified as to with fat ☛ 32 (Low)

Mushrooms—cooked, from canned, with fat ☞ 32 (Low)

Mushrooms—cooked, from canned, without fat ☞ 32 (Low)

Mushrooms—cooked, from fresh, Not Specified as to with fat ☞ 32 (Low)

Mushrooms—cooked, from fresh, with fat ☞ 32 (Low)

Mushrooms—cooked, from fresh, without fat ☞ 32 (Low)

Mushrooms—cooked, from frozen, Not Specified as to with fat ☞ 32 (Low)

Mushrooms—cooked, from frozen, with fat ☞ 32 (Low)

Mushrooms—cooked, Not Specified as to form, Not Specified as to with fat ☞ 32 (Low)

Mushrooms—cooked, Not Specified as to form, with fat ☞ 32 (Low)

Mushrooms—cooked, Not Specified as to form, without fat ☞ 32 (Low)

Mushrooms—pickled ☞ 32 (Low)

Mushrooms—raw ☞ 32 (Low)

Mustard greeNot Specified—cooked, from canned, without fat ☞ 32 (Low)

Mustard greeNot Specified—cooked, from fresh, without fat ☞ 32 (Low)

Mustard greeNot Specified—cooked, from frozen, without fat ☞ 32 (Low)

Mustard greeNot Specified—cooked, Not Specified as to form, without fat ☞ 32 (Low)

Mustard pickles ☞ 32 (Low)

🟤 Okra—cooked, from canned, with fat ☛ 32 (Low)

🟤 Okra—cooked, from canned, without fat ☛ 32 (Low)

🟤 Okra—cooked, from fresh, Not Specified as to with fat ☛ 32 (Low)

🟤 Okra—cooked, from fresh, with fat ☛ 32 (Low)

🟤 Okra—cooked, from fresh, without fat ☛ 32 (Low)

🟤 Okra—cooked, from frozen, Not Specified as to with fat ☛ 32 (Low)

🟤 Okra—cooked, from frozen, with fat ☛ 32 (Low)

🟤 Okra—cooked, from frozen, without fat ☛ 32 (Low)

🟤 Okra—cooked, Not Specified as to form, Not Specified as to with fat ☛ 32 (Low)

🟤 Okra—cooked, Not Specified as to form, with fat ☛ 32 (Low)

🟤 Okra—cooked, Not Specified as to form, without fat ☛ 32 (Low)

🟤 Okra—pickled ☛ 32 (Low)

🟤 Olives—black ☛ 50 (Low)

🟤 Olives—green ☛ 50 (Low)

🟤 Olives—green, stuffed ☛ 50 (Low)

🟤 Olives—NFS ☛ 50 (Low)

🟤 Onion, young green, cooked, Not Specified as to form, Not Specified as to with fat ☛ 32 (Low)

🟤 OnioNot Specified—mature, cooked, from fresh, without fat ☛ 32 (Low)

🟤 OnioNot Specified—mature, cooked, from frozen, without fat ☛ 32 (Low)

OnioNot Specified—mature, cooked, Not Specified as to form, without fat ☞ 32 (Low)

OnioNot Specified—mature, raw ☞ 32 (Low)

OnioNot Specified—pearl, cooked, from canned ☞ 32 (Low)

OnioNot Specified—pearl, cooked, from fresh ☞ 32 (Low)

OnioNot Specified—pearl, cooked, Not Specified as to form ☞ 32 (Low)

OnioNot Specified—young green, cooked, from fresh, without fat ☞ 32 (Low)

OnioNot Specified—young green, cooked, Not Specified as to form, without fat ☞ 32 (Low)

OnioNot Specifiedcyoung green, raw ☞ 32 (Low)

Palm hearts—cooked without fat ☞ 32 (Low)

Parsley—cooked without fat ☞ 32 (Low)

Parsley—raw ☞ 32 (Low)

Parsnips—cooked, with fat ☞ 97 (High)

Parsnips—cooked, without fat ☞ 97 (High)

Peas and Carrots—canned, low sodium, without fat ☞ 48 (Low)

Peas and Carrots—cooked, from canned, without fat ☞ 48 (Low)

Peas and Carrots—cooked, from fresh, without fat ☞ 48 (Low)

Peas and Carrots—cooked, from frozen, without fat ☞ 48 (Low)

Peas and Carrots—cooked, Not Specified as to form, without fat ☞ 48 (Low)

Peas and corn—cooked, without fat ☞ 51 (Low)

Peas and OnioNot Specified—cooked, without fat ☞ 40 (Low)

- Peas and potatoes—cooked, without fat ☞ 63 (Medium)

- Peas with Mushrooms—cooked, without fat ☞ 47 (Low)

- Peas, cowpeas—cooked, from canned, without fat ☞ 42 (Low)

- Peas, cowpeas—cooked, from fresh, without fat ☞ 42 (Low)

- Peas, cowpeas—cooked, from frozen, without fat ☞ 42 (Low)

- Peas, cowpeas—cooked, Not Specified as to form, without fat ☞ 42 (Low)

- Peas, green—canned, low sodium, without fat ☞ 48 (Low)

- Peas, green—cooked, from canned, without fat ☞ 48 (Low)

- Peas, green—cooked, from fresh, without fat ☞ 48 (Low)

- Peas, green—cooked, from frozen, without fat ☞ 48 (Low)

- Peas, green—cooked, Not Specified as to form, without fat ☞ 48 (Low)

- Peas, green—raw ☞ 48 (Low)

- Pepper—green, cooked, without fat ☞ 32 (Low)

- Pepper—hot chili, raw ☞ 32 (Low)

- Pepper—hot, cooked, from canned, Not Specified as to with fat ☞ 32 (Low)

- Pepper—hot, cooked, from canned, with fat ☞ 32 (Low)

- Pepper—hot, cooked, from canned, without fat ☞ 32 (Low)

- Pepper—hot, cooked, from fresh, Not Specified as to with fat ☞ 32 (Low)

- Pepper—hot, cooked, from fresh, with fat ☞ 32 (Low)

- Pepper—hot, cooked, from fresh, without fat ☞ 32 (Low)

- Pepper—hot, cooked, from frozen, without fat ☞ 32 (Low)

Pepper—hot, cooked, Not Specified as to form, Not Specified as to with fat ☞ 32 (Low)

Pepper—hot, cooked, Not Specified as to form, with fat ☞ 32 (Low)

Pepper—hot, cooked, Not Specified as to form, without fat ☞ 32 (Low)

Pepper—hot, pickled ☞ 32 (Low)

Pepper—pickled ☞ 32 (Low)

Pepper—poblano, raw ☞ 32 (Low)

Pepper—raw, NFS ☞ 32 (Low)

Pepper—red, cooked, without fat ☞ 32 (Low)

Pepper—Serrano, raw ☞ 32 (Low)

Pepper—sweet, green, raw ☞ 32 (Low)

Pepper—sweet, red, raw ☞ 32 (Low)

Pigeon peas—cooked, Not Specified as to form, without fat ☞ 22 (Low)

Pimiento ☞ 32 (Low)

Pumpkin—cooked, from canned, without fat ☞ 75 (High)

Pumpkin—cooked, from fresh, with fat ☞ 75 (High)

Pumpkin—cooked, from fresh, without fat ☞ 75 (High)

Pumpkin—cooked, Not Specified as to form, without fat ☞ 75 (High)

Radish—common, raw ☞ 32 (Low)

Radish—Japanese (daikon), cooked, without fat ☞ 32 (Low)

Radish—raw ☞ 32 (Low)

Radishes—pickled, Hawaiian style ☛ 32 (Low)

Recaito (little coriander) ☛ 32 (Low)

Rutabaga—cooked, with fat ☛ 72 (High)

Rutabaga—cooked, without fat ☛ 72 (High)

Salsa—NFS ☛ 38 (Low)

Salsa—red, cooked, homemade ☛ 38 (Low)

Salsa—red, cooked, not homemade ☛ 38 (Low)

Salsa—red, uncooked ☛ 38 (Low)

Sauerkraut—canned ☛ 32 (Low)

Sauerkraut—cooked, Not Specified as to with fat ☛ 32 (Low)

Sauerkraut—cooked, with fat ☛ 32 (Low)

Sauerkraut—cooked, without fat ☛ 32 (Low)

Seaweed—dried ☛ 32 (Low)

Seaweed—prepared with soy sauce ☛ 32 (Low)

Seaweed—raw ☛ 32 (Low)

Snowpea—cooked, from fresh, without fat ☛ 32 (Low)

Snowpea—cooked, from frozen, without fat ☛ 32 (Low)

Snowpea—cooked, Not Specified as to form, without fat ☛ 32 (Low)

Snowpeas raw ☛ 32 (Low)

Spinach—cooked, from canned, without fat ☛ 32 (Low)

Spinach—cooked, from fresh, without fat ☛ 32 (Low)

Spinach—cooked, from frozen, without fat ☛ 32 (Low)

Spinach—cooked, Not Specified as to form, without fat ☛

32 (Low)

⬤ Spinach—raw ☞ 32 (Low)

⬤ Sprouts ☞ 32 (Low)

⬤ Squash, spaghetti—cooked, Not Specified as to with fat ☞ 32 (Low)

⬤ Squash, spaghetti—cooked, without fat ☞ 32 (Low)

⬤ Squash, summer—and OnioNot Specified—cooked, without fat ☞ 32 (Low)

⬤ Squash, summer—cooked, from canned, Not Specified as to with fat ☞ 32 (Low)

⬤ Squash, summer—cooked, from canned, with fat ☞ 32 (Low)

⬤ Squash, summer—cooked, from canned, without fat ☞ 32 (Low)

⬤ Squash, summer—cooked, from fresh, Not Specified as to with fat ☞ 32 (Low)

⬤ Squash, summer—cooked, from fresh, with fat ☞ 32 (Low)

⬤ Squash, summer—cooked, from fresh, without fat ☞ 32 (Low)

⬤ Squash, summer—cooked, from frozen, with fat ☞ 32 (Low)

⬤ Squash, summer—cooked, from frozen, without fat ☞ 32 (Low)

⬤ Squash, summer—cooked, Not Specified as to form, Not Specified as to with fat ☞ 32 (Low)

⬤ Squash, summer—cooked, Not Specified as to form, with fat ☞ 32 (Low)

⬤ Squash, summer—cooked, Not Specified as to form, without fat ☞ 32 (Low)

⬤ Squash, summer—from fresh, creamed ☞ 29 (Low)

⬤ Squash, summer—green, raw ☞ 32 (Low)

Squash, summer—yellow, raw ☛ 32 (Low)

Squash, winter—baked, fat and sugar added in cooking ☛ 71 (High)

Squash, winter—baked, no fat or sugar added in cooking ☛ 75 (High)

Squash, winter—baked, no with fat, sugar added in cooking ☛ 71 (High)

Squash, winter—baked, Not Specified as to fat or sugar added in cooking ☛ 71 (High)

Squash, winter—baked, with fat, no sugar added in cooking ☛ 75 (High)

Squash, winter—mashed, fat and sugar added in cooking ☛ 71 (High)

Squash, winter—mashed, no fat or sugar added in cooking ☛ 75 (High)

Squash, winter—mashed, Not Specified as to fat or sugar added in cooking ☛ 75 (High)

Squash, winter—mashed, with fat, no sugar added in cooking ☛ 75 (High)

Sweetpotato leaves,—cooked, without fat ☛ 32 (Low)

Sweetpotato with fruit ☛ 53 (Low)

Sweetpotato—baked, peel eaten, without fat ☛ 61 (Medium)

Sweetpotato—baked, peel not eaten, without fat ☛ 61 (Medium)

Sweetpotato—boiled, with peel, without fat ☛ 61 (Medium)

Sweetpotato—boiled, without peel, without fat ☛ 61 (Medium)

Sweetpotato—canned in syrup ☛ 61 (Medium)

Sweetpotato—canned without syrup ☞ 61 (Medium)

Sweetpotato—canned, Not Specified as to syrup ☞ 61 (Medium)

Tannier—cooked ☞ 32 (Low)

Taro leaves—cooked, without fat ☞ 32 (Low)

Taro—baked ☞ 55 (Low)

Tomato and corn—cooked, without fat ☞ 50 (Low)

Tomato and Okra—cooked, without fat ☞ 35 (Low)

Tomato and onion—cooked, Not Specified as to with fat ☞ 35 (Low)

Tomato and onion, cooked, without fat ☞ 35 (Low)

Tomato catsup ☞ 38 (Low)

Tomato chili sauce ☞ 38 (Low)

Tomato paste ☞ 38 (Low)

Tomato relish ☞ 32 (Low)

Tomato—green, pickled ☞ 32 (Low)

Tomato—green, raw ☞ 38 (Low)

Tomato—raw ☞ 38 (Low)

Turnip greeNot Specified—cooked, from canned, without fat ☞ 32 (Low)

Turnip greeNot Specified—cooked, from fresh, without fat ☞ 32 (Low)

Turnip greeNot Specified—cooked, from frozen, without fat ☞ 32 (Low)

Turnip greeNot Specified—cooked, Not Specified as to form, without fat ☞ 32 (Low)

Turnip greeNot Specified—with roots, cooked, from frozen, without fat 🖙 32 (Low)

Turnip—cooked, from fresh, Not Specified as to with fat 🖙 72 (High)

Turnip—cooked, from fresh, with fat 🖙 72 (High)

Turnip—cooked, from fresh, without fat 🖙 72 (High)

Turnip—cooked, Not Specified as to form, with fat 🖙 72 (High)

Turnip—cooked, Not Specified as to form, without fat 🖙 72 (High)

Turnip—from fresh, creamed 🖙 40 (Low)

Turnip—raw 🖙 72 (High)

Vegetable relish 🖙 32 (Low)

Vegetables—cooked, Not Specified as to with fat, average value 🖙 43 (Low)

Vegetables—cooked, without fat, average value 🖙 43 (Low)

Vegetables—pickled 🖙 32 (Low)

Vegetables, stew type—potatoes, Carrots, OnioNot Specified and celery, cooked, without fat 🖙 62 (Medium)

Water chestnut 🖙 32 (Low)

Watercress—raw 🖙 32 (Low)

White potato 🖙 66 (Medium)

White potato—baked, peel eaten, without fat 🖙 73 (High)

White potato—baked, peel not eaten 🖙 73 (High)

White potato—boiled, with peel, without fat 🖙 66 (Medium)

White potato—boiled, without peel, canned, low sodium, without fat 🖙 63 (Medium)

White potato—boiled, without peel, without fat ☞ 66 (Medium)

White potato—french fries, breaded or battered ☞ 75 (High)

White potato—french fries, from fresh, deep fried ☞ 75 (High)

White potato—french fries, from frozen, deep fried ☞ 75 (High)

White potato—french fries, from frozen, oven baked ☞ 75 (High)

White potato—french fries, Not Specified as to from fresh or frozen ☞ 75 (High)

White potato—from complete dry mix, mashed, made with water ☞ 85 (High)

White potato—from dry, mashed, made with milk, no fat ☞ 85 (High)

White potato—from fresh, mashed, made with milk ☞ 79 (High)

White potato—from fresh, mashed, not made with milk or fat ☞ 79 (High)

White potato—hash brown, from dry mix ☞ 75 (High)

White potato—hash brown, from fresh ☞ 75 (High)

White potato—hash brown, from frozen ☞ 75 (High)

White potato—hash brown, Not Specified as to from fresh, frozen, or dry mix ☞ 75 (High)

White potato—hash brown, with cheese ☞ 75 (High)

White potato—home fries ☞ 75 (High)

White potato—roasted, without fat ☞ 73 (High)

Winter melon—cooked ☞ 32 (Low)

Yam—cooked ☞ 37 (Low)

Zucchini—cooked, tomato sauce, without fat ☞ 35 (Low)

HEALTH AND NUTRITION WEBSITES

American Diabetes Association

(www.diabetes.org)

American Heart Association

(www.americanheart.org)

Centers for Disease Control and Prevention

(www.cdc.gov/healthyweight)

Cooking Light

(www.cookinglight.com)

Eating Well

(www.eatingwell.com)

eMedicine Health

(www.emedicinehealth.com)

Fruits and Vegetables Matter

(www.fruitsandveggiesmatter.gov)

Health

(www.health.com)

Hormone Foundation

(www.hormone.org)

National Heart, Lung, Blood Institute

(www.nhlbi.nih.gov)

National Institute on Aging

(www.nia.nih.gov)

National Institutes of Health

(http://health.nih.gov)

Nutrition.gov (www.nutrition.gov)

Prevention (www.prevention.com)

Made in the USA
Monee, IL
14 August 2022

11641097R00167